THE DINOSAUR TAMER

And Other Stories for Children with Diabetes

By

Marcia Levine Mazur,

Peter Banks,
and Andrew Keegan

 American Diabetes Association.

Publisher	Susan H. Lau
Editorial Director	Peter Banks
Editor and designer	Sherrye Landrum
Cover art	Elizabeth Wolfe
Cover design	Rene Boudreau
Illustrations	Patty Walsh
Desktop publishing	Stacey Wages
Production Director	Carolyn Segree

Printed in the United States of America

American Diabetes Association, Inc.
1660 Duke Street
Alexandria, VA 22314

Library of Congress Cataloging-in-Publication Data
Mazur, Marcia Levine, 1933-
The dinosaur tamer and other stories for children with diabetes/by Marcia Levine Mazur, Peter Banks, and Andrew Keegan.
p.   cm.
Summary: A collection of twenty-five stories portraying children with diabetes doing usual things such as expressing their emotions, coping with difficulties, and having fun.
ISBN 0-945448-58-9; $9.95
      1. Diabetes—Juvenile fiction. 2. Children's stories, American. [1. Diabetes—Fiction. 2. Diseases—Fiction. 3. Short stories]
      I. Banks, Peter, 1955- . II. Keegan, Andrew, 1949- .
      II. Mazur, Marcia   III. Title
PZ5.M543Di 1995
[Fic]—dc20   95-43126
                                        CIP
                                        AC

Table of Contents

Diabetes is New to Me

Sometimes You Need A Little Magic

Preface to Families

The American Diabetes Association Kid's Corner stories, a new genre of health education literature, began in 1988. These enjoyable and imaginative fictional stories are about children with diabetes, in family life, at school, and at play. They are designed to help children learn about and sustain their interest in diabetes. The stories are interwoven with ideas about positive ways to cope with concerns and adjustment issues common to children everywhere. The stories collected here first appeared in *Diabetes Forecast* magazine.

As a former Kid's Corner advisor, I helped to generate ideas for the stories by drawing on my social work experience in the diabetes program at Children's National Medical Center, Washington, DC. The children and families often saw their own experiences reflected in the stories.

Children with diabetes face situations, both real and imagined, that can cause them emotional distress. Identifying with story characters allows them to see their own situations and new possibilities more clearly. They can imagine being braver and more confident, like the boy in *The Red Baseball Cap*. They might master their feelings about the unfairness of having diabetes, as did the child in *Why Me?* Families can learn about the importance of working together, as is highlighted in *Please Listen, Dad. . . .*

What children absorb when they read these stories may change from one time to another. It is recommended that you read the stories, too, so that you are familiar with them and can talk comfortably about ideas contained in them with your children.

This collection of stories is at once delightful and educational. It also emphasizes the strengths and potential for growth within each child and family.

Sandra F. Epstein, LCSW-C

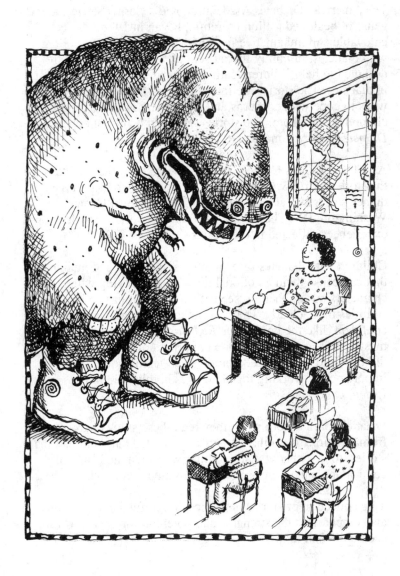

The Dinosaur Tamer

by Peter Banks

Every time he went to Dr. Cavanaugh's office, Danny Littleton turned into a dinosaur. He wasn't just any dinosaur. Who, after all, would want to be a Brontosaurus, fat and slow? Or a Stegosaurus, with all those rattling plates on its back. No, Danny always turned into one special dinosaur—a Tyrannosaurus, strong and fearless, the king of the dinosaurs.

Of course, his mother just thought he was daydreaming again. Grown-ups always said that he daydreamed too much.

Once, his teacher Mrs. Parker had called his mother to say that Danny was distractible in class. He'd had to look up that word, distractible. It meant he wasn't paying attention.

Of course, he couldn't make anyone understand. How could a grown-up understand about a Tyrannosaurus? A Tyrannosaurus couldn't just stop in his tracks and answer a question like what was the capitol of Illinois or how much was 9 times 7.

A Tyrannosaurus also didn't have time to be afraid of anything. If he had diabetes, a Tyrannosaurus would never be afraid to tell Mary Ellen Sullivan to stop saying those things about him.

Mary Ellen was a girl Danny had liked until the day he overheard her talking about him at recess.

"Danny's got diabetes," she said to a bunch of other kids. "That means he's sick, and he's got to take shots and eat special food and stuff."

It made Danny mad that all the kids thought he was sick. He wasn't sick! He just had diabetes, that was all. He played baseball and basketball just like the other kids.

He wanted to go right up to Mary Ellen and tell her to stop telling kids he was sick. But every time he thought about doing that, he got scared and didn't do it.

And so, last Monday, when Danny actually had come down with the flu and felt bad, he hadn't told his Mom or Dad. He knew that he was supposed to. Dr. Cavanaugh said all the time that if he felt sick, it was important to tell. But Danny couldn't do it. He wasn't going to let everybody in his class think Mary Ellen was right.

But that's what they thought anyway, now, because after he had gotten to school he had felt terrible. Mrs. Parker had noticed how he looked and sent him to the school nurse. When the nurse pulled the thermometer from his mouth and said "102—guess you get to go home," Danny starting crying and couldn't stop.

Partly, it was because he felt so sick. But even more it was because now everyone would know he wasn't strong and fearless but just Danny Littleton, who was sick with diabetes just the way Mary Ellen said.

Thinking about it now, sitting beside his Mom in the waiting room, he turned into a Tyrannosaurus again. He stamped around the room, hooking his big clawed feet into

Dr. Cavanaugh's gray carpet. He felt as if he were 100 feet high. The people in the waiting room looked as small as the little goldfish in Dr. Cavanaugh's aquarium.

He was just about to throw his head back and roar when he heard someone calling, "Danny, Danny." His mother was tugging at his sleeve. "Danny, stop daydreaming. The doctor is ready to see you." Sure enough, a nurse was holding a door open for him.

His mother started to get up, but Danny asked her to stay. "You come to the doctor's office after he looks at me," he said. There was no way you could be strong and fearless when your Mom was always following you like you were a baby.

The nurse took Danny to a little examining room. "Dr. Cavanaugh isn't here today, so you'll see Dr. Wilson. He works with Dr. Cavanaugh now. I think you'll like him a lot. He'll be in in a minute." She shut the door behind her.

Danny slumped down in the plastic chair. It didn't matter what doctor he saw. They would all say the same thing: He should always tell his Mom and Dad when he felt sick because his blood sugar could go too high.

Danny stood up and started to walk back and forth in the little room, a Tyrannosaurus again. He could see himself marching through the forest and people scrambling to get out of his way.

Just as he had started to do before, he put his head back and roared—but quietly, so no one did hear.

But someone did hear, because just at that moment, the door opened. "Hi, I'm Dr. Wilson," a man's voice said. "That was quite a roar." Danny turned around. He could feel his face getting hot and red.

Then he noticed that the doctor was in a wheelchair.

3

Dr. Wilson pushed into the room and closed the door behind him. "I roar myself, sometimes. It makes me feel better," Dr. Wilson said.

Danny laughed. He couldn't picture a doctor roaring. He also couldn't picture a doctor in a wheelchair.

"How come you're in a wheelchair?" Danny asked.

"I was in an accident when I was a teenager."

"Are you going to get better?" Danny asked.

"I'm not going to walk again if that's what you mean," Dr. Wilson said.

"Oh," Danny said. He couldn't think of what else to say.

"Danny," Dr. Wilson rolled his chair closer, "I'm going to check you to make sure that infection's gone, but I want to talk to you a minute first. Your Mom said that you didn't tell her you had the flu. How come?"

Danny looked at the floor. He wished he could turn into a Tyrannosaurus now, but this time he stayed just Danny Littleton. He looked up at Dr. Wilson. "I was scared," he said.

"What were you scared of?"

He bit his lower lip. "All the kids at school think I'm sick because I have diabetes. I wanted to show them I'm not."

Now Dr. Wilson would probably be mad at him and tell him he was dumb to forget to tell. But instead he said, "Danny, do you think I'm sick?"

Danny looked down at Dr. Wilson's wheelchair. "Well, yes—I mean no—you're not like sick. Not like the flu or a cold or anything like that."

Dr. Wilson nodded. "That's right. I'm not sick, I just can't walk anymore," he said. "And you're not sick, either.

Your body just doesn't use food like it used to, so it needs some help from shots. But having diabetes doesn't mean you're sick. A cold, a flu, a stomach ache—that's sick. But diabetes is normal for you."

"But that's what Mary Ellen said," Danny replied. "She told everybody."

"Then Mary Ellen doesn't know very much about diabetes, does she?" Dr. Wilson said. "Maybe you could tell her and the other kids what diabetes really means."

"I can't," Danny said. "She'd laugh. I'd be too afraid." Danny slumped down more in his chair. He wasn't like a Tyrannosaurus at all.

"You know, after I had my accident, I was really afraid, too," Dr. Wilson said. "I had always wanted to be a doctor, but a lot of people told me I couldn't be one. 'You'd better just forget it,' they said."

"What did you do?" Danny asked.

"Well I had kind of a secret way of making myself feel brave again," said Dr. Wilson. "In high school, I was a diver. What made me feel really strong was diving—being weightless, over the water just like a bird. Sometimes I thought I could really fly."

"After my accident, I couldn't dive anymore. But I could remember what diving felt like. And every time I felt scared, I just pictured myself in a dive."

Dr. Wilson looked at Danny. "I wonder if you have something like that you like to think about that makes you feel strong." He smiled. "Maybe sometimes you feel like some animal that roared."

"A Tyrannosaurus!" Danny said.

Dr. Wilson nodded and smiled again. "Well, Mr. Tyrannosaurus," he said. "I'll bet you're not afraid of anything."

"Nope." Danny smiled.

"So if you get a cold or a flu you won't be afraid to tell your Mom and Dad."

"Nope," And Danny knew it was true.

"And I'll bet you won't be afraid to tell this Mary Ellen what's what next time she says something dumb about diabetes."

Danny paused. He didn't smile this time. "Nope," he said finally. But he wasn't sure if he could do it, Tyrannosaurus or not.

The next day, he told himself, was the day to tell Mary Ellen. But three o'clock came, and the bell rang, and he just went home.

That happened the next day and the day after and the day after that. Danny decided he would just forget about it—he would let everybody think he was sick.

One day, though, during story hour, when everyone was supposed to tell a story, he had an idea. His hand shot up to be called on before he even knew what he was doing. He couldn't face Mary Ellen alone, but maybe he could tell the class about him.

As soon as he got to the front of the class, though, he started to see what a mistake he had made. His hands started to feel cold and sweaty. Everyone was staring at him. He would probably say something dumb, and Mary Ellen Sullivan would laugh out loud.

Then he remembered what Dr. Wilson had said. What would a Tyrannosaurus do? As soon as he thought that, Danny felt himself looking down at everybody. He was Danny the Tyrannosaurus, staring down at Mrs. Parker's fifth-grade class. Everybody seemed as little as ants.

Then he started to talk, in a big, strong voice that he hardly knew as his own voice. "I have diabetes," he began. "But that doesn't mean I'm sick. I can do all kinds of things."

"Why Me?"

by Andrew Keegan

Why me? Robert must have asked himself that question 10,000 times since that day three months ago when Dr. Conforti told him, and his mom and dad, that he had diabetes.

What did he do to deserve diabetes? He'd always gotten passing grades in school. He was a good teammate to all his friends on the baseball team. And he was always—well, almost always—nice to his brother Sam. (And it wasn't exactly easy having a little brother.) Getting diabetes just wasn't fair.

It was almost as if someone had reached out, tapped him on the shoulder, and said, "You're it." Only this wasn't a game—it was real, and pretty awful.

Since the day he was diagnosed with diabetes, Robert had wanted to find out why he was the one who ended up with it. So he went to his father. If any one could understand diabetes, it was his dad. That night in the hospital, when Robert felt so sick and scared, it was his father's hand on his shoulder that kept Robert from feeling that diabetes was a towering monster ready to swallow him up.

But later, when he asked his father why he got diabetes, his father really didn't have an answer. He just said something about it not being Robert's fault. The truth was, his father didn't know. It scared Robert a little to think that his dad—who knew baseball statistics back to the time when the Dodgers were in Brooklyn and a team called the Senators played in Washington—just couldn't answer his questions.

But Dr. Conforti would be different—it was her job to know. He would ask her.

His chance came during an office visit the next week. After the exam and blood test, Robert got up his courage. He fired off three questions in a row to Dr. Conforti, boom, boom, boom: "Why did I get diabetes? What did I do? Why me?"

"Well, Robert, those are not easy questions," Dr. Conforti told him.

"Sometimes a person's body just stops making insulin. Insulin helps our bodies turn food into energy. Without insulin, our bodies don't work well. That's why you felt sick before we knew what was wrong, and why you felt better after we gave you an insulin injection.

"But," she admitted, "even doctors and scientists don't completely understand why some people get diabetes and others don't. We're working on it, though. Some day we hope to find the answers. The important thing now is for you to take care of yourself."

"So even scientists don't have an answer!" Robert thought to himself.

He was grateful to Dr. Conforti for taking the time to explain how diabetes worked. But Robert was more interested in finding out why he got it. He still felt like he had been picked out of the crowd. He still felt alone.

Robert wasn't ready to give up his search for an answer yet, but who else could he ask? He thought of all the adults he knew, and decided to try his parish priest—and baseball coach—Father Ryan. Maybe he would know.

After Sunday Mass, Robert went up to Father Ryan, who was greeting the churchgoers as they filed out through the main door.

"Can I ask you a question, Father?" Robert asked.

"Give me a few moments here, Bobby, and then we'll talk," Father Ryan said.

After the last group of parishioners had left the church, Father Ryan came over to Robert and asked him what was on his mind.

"Nothing much, Father. I've just been wondering," Robert said.

"Wondering about what?"

"Father, why'd I have to get diabetes?" Robert asked. "What did I do? Why me?"

Father Ryan thought for a moment, rubbed his chin a bit, and then spoke.

"A lot of things happen in this world, Bobby, and not all of them make sense," Father Ryan said.

"Think of it this way. Life is like a beautiful tapestry woven out of all the colors of the rainbow: reds, greens, blues, silver, gold. The threads are our thoughts, dreams, even the things that make us angry or sad. We can't see the overall pattern or figure out how it all fits together, but God can. And every thread you weave is important to Him.

"Bad things sometimes happen," Father Ryan said, "but when they do, we believe that God is always there for us, to help us and to share His love."

For the next few days Robert found himself thinking about what Father Ryan had said. It made a lot of sense. After all, there were hundreds of things he didn't under-stand, like the pull of magnets, how rainbows suddenly appear after it rains, or why balls drop down and not up when you let them go. A lot of things don't make perfect sense, but they happen anyway. And it all kind of fits together, in a way.

So, instead of worrying about the "whys," Robert concentrated on dealing with the everyday routine of finger pricks, injections, and meal plans. "I guess you can get used to anything," he thought.

Saturday

Robert couldn't wait for Saturday to arrive. He was scheduled to play baseball that afternoon, but first, his Dad had promised to take the whole family on a trip to the old downtown section of the city. Robert loved the shops, the toy stores, and especially talking to Old Man Jacobs, the little old man who ran Jacobs' Cleaners.

In the past few years, Mr. Jacobs had opened up a whole new world to Robert: The World of Baseball in the 1920s and 1930s. He'd seen all the legends: Babe Ruth, Ty Cobb, Walter Johnson. Tacked to his walls were yellowed newspaper clippings and glossy photographs of all the greats, Mr. Jacobs' own Hall of Fame. Robert loved talking baseball with him.

Once in town, Robert's family went off in different directions; his mother went with Sam to buy him a new pair of sneakers, and Robert and his father ducked into and out of the shops along Main Street. Finally they reached the sign that said, "Jacob's Cleaners."

They opened the door, making a little bell jingle. Mr. Jacobs greeted them both with a big hello.

"Bernie, I've got to run across the street to buy some greeting cards," Robert's father said. "Robert would like to stay here with you for a few minutes. Is that OK?"

"Sure, sure, take your time," Mr. Jacobs answered. Robert's father nodded and closed the door behind him.

"So tell me," Mr. Jacobs said, looking down at Robert, "How are you doing?"

"OK, I guess," Robert answered.

"You guess. You don't know?" Mr. Jacobs asked.

"Here, I've got just the thing for you," he said, reaching under the counter with one hand and lifting a candy bar over his head like a Fourth of July sparkler. "Have some chocolate. You'll feel better."

"No I won't. That's the problem," Robert said. "I've already had lunch and I can't eat that candy bar because the doctor told me I have diabetes. . .I hate it."

"So you can't have a little piece of candy!" Mr. Jacobs said. "What s the big deal? What's so bad about diabetes?"

"What's so bad?" Robert couldn't believe that anyone would even ask him that question.

"Here's what's so bad," Robert said. "Number one, I have to prick my fingers every day. Then I have to get shots. And I can't even eat the things I want to most of the time, like that candy bar. It's not fair—no one else on my baseball team, nobody else I even know, has to do any of that. Why should I? Why me?"

Mr. Jacobs looked right at Robert. "You know something? You're right. It's not fair. You got a rotten deal."

Robert was a little surprised to hear him say this. It wasn't what he expected.

Mr. Jacobs walked slowly over to the wall and untacked a photograph. "Do you recognize this fellow?" he asked.

Robert studied the face. "I think it's Lou Gehrig," he said. Robert knew his baseball history.

"And what do you know about him?"

"I know he was a teammate of Babe Ruth. And I know

he held the record for playing the most games in a row—
until Cal Ripkin broke it."

"Right you are, Robert. They called him the Iron
Horse, because he was so indestructible. Do you know
how his streak ended?"

"No," Robert said.

"It ended because he took himself out of a game. He
was sick. In fact, he was dying."

"They held a special day for him in Yankee Stadium on
July 4, 1939. I'll never forget it. I was there. And do you
know what Gehrig, who was so sick his legs were shaking,
told the crowd? He said, 'Today I consider myself the
luckiest man on the face of the earth.'"

"Why'd he say he was lucky?" Robert asked. "His
streak was over, and he was sick. What's so lucky about
that?"

Mr. Jacobs thought for a moment before answering,
and when he did, he chose his words very carefully. "He
was lucky, Robert, because he had love.

"That day Gehrig didn't talk about his streak, or his
home runs, or any of his accomplishments," Mr. Jacobs
said. "He thanked the fans for their kindness and encourage-
ment. He thanked all the people he met during his years in
the game, even the groundskeepers. He thanked his mother
and his father and his wife. He thanked everyone who loved
him. In one afternoon, he tried to give back all the love that
people had been giving to him over the years.

"That's why he considered himself the luckiest man on
earth: He loved people, and people loved him."

Just as Mr. Jacobs finished his story, the little bell to
his shop rang again, and Robert's dad pushed through.

"This boy been giving you any trouble, Bernie?" he

13

said, laughing. "Maybe he needs to be pressed and fold-ed." He pulled Robert's baseball cap over his eyes.

Robert pushed his cap back to the top of his head and looked hard at his dad, who kept an arm on his shoulder. It didn't seem so important anymore that his father couldn't answer why Robert got diabetes. No one could, just the way no one could answer why Lou Gehrig got sick.

Maybe the "why" didn't matter that much. What did matter was that his father and mother were always there when diabetes seemed so scary, just the way people in the stadium had cheered Gehrig on.

"Gotta run. Take care, Bernie," Robert's dad said.

"You too," Mr. Jacobs replied. Then the old man bent down and offered his hand to Robert. "I'm sorry to hear that you have diabetes, Robert," he said, shaking Robert's hand. "Come by anytime, and we'll talk some more."

"It's a deal. See ya next time!" Robert said. Then he and his dad walked out the door of the dimly lit shop and into the blinding sunlight of the bright morning.

Down the street, Robert could see his mother and Sam leaning against the family car. Both turned at the same moment, and waved at him. His dad tapped him lightly on the top of his head. "Time to get you home—we've got to get ready for the ballgame, son," he said.

At that moment, something like a wave rippled through Robert's body from his toes to his head, a feeling deep inside that he hadn't felt in quite awhile. Maybe it was having his family all together, or Mr. Jacobs' story, or the baseball game. Maybe it was the sun shining in his face. Or maybe it was all of these things coming together all at once. He didn't know. He didn't care.

He was happy.

The Diamond Bracelet

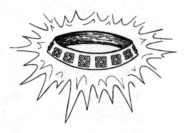

by Marcia Levine Mazur

Still wearing our Halloween clown costumes, my best
friend, Kim, and I ran into my kitchen and emptied our
trick-or-treat bags onto the table.

We'd just come back from collecting Halloween good-
ies on 144th Street. My Mom had been with us all
evening, of course, but she'd waited on the sidewalk while
we knocked on all the doors.

Kim and I were glad she was there this year because
this Halloween had been really scary. There was a big jewelry store robbery about ten blocks away the night before,
and the thief hadn't been caught yet.

We weren't thinking about that, though, when we started
picking through our bags. We just wanted to see our loot.

There was the usual stuff, miniature chocolate bars—
Mrs. Kinghorn gave those just like she does every year.
And hard candies in colored wrappers—they were from
the Picker's. Small bags of peanuts had to be from Jennie
Peiros. Her husband always brought peanuts home. I think
he worked in a peanut store or something.

There was an apple and a couple of nickels and a few

loose raisins that made everything sticky.

But there was one thing more in my bag—a diamond bracelet.

"Wow!" Kim grabbed it from me and held it up to the light. "Who gave you this, Leslie?"

"I don't know," I said in a whisper, pulling it back. "I can't even imagine."

We looked at each other and we both had the same thought, but Kim said it first. "It's from the jewel robbery."

I circled the sparkly chain around my wrist and smiled at it. I didn't know if it was from the robbery or not. But I was sure it was made of real diamonds. It looked so grown-up, not like any of the junk in my own small pink jewelry box with the ballerina on top.

'Wait, I know," Kim said. "Junior Tomkin put that bracelet in your bag. He was probably in on the robbery. I always thought there was something funny about him." Kim had a great imagination.

"Junior Tomkin? Don't be silly," I said.

"OK, Leslie," she bit her lip, thinking. "Suppose it s not from the jewel robbery. Maybe it's from Mrs. Nelson's baby. Remember how the baby grabbed the bag and Mrs. Nelson had to pull it away?"

"But where would a baby get a diamond bracelet?"

"My cousin's baby got her wedding ring and threw it into the dishwasher," Kim told me. "Babies get a hold of a lot of things."

She might have something there, I decided. The Nelson's baby *had* played with the bag.

But Kim was already working on another idea. "No. It was Old Lady Dishler." She gave a little shiver. "I'm glad I waited with your mom when you went there. She's weird."

16

"Oh, Kim," I said, kind of annoyed. "Just because she is in a wheelchair? Besides, she was nice. She asked me what kind of candy I wanted. I told her I'd rather have something else since I couldn't eat much candy because I had diabetes. And you know what she did then?"

"I can't imagine," Kim said sarcastically.

"She patted me on the head and told me to take good care of myself."

Kim shrugged. "Well, Leslie, who wants an old lady patting you on the head anyway?"

Then Kim asked the question I'd been asking myself. "You going to tell your mom and dad about the bracelet?"

"I guess," I said, "in a day or two."

I knew I should tell Mom and Dad right away. Maybe even the police. But I wanted to see if I could figure out this mystery by myself. Who could have dropped a diamond bracelet in my Halloween bag? And why?

Mom came into the kitchen then and real fast I stuffed the bracelet and everything else back into my bag.

"Get anything good?" she asked.

I didn't answer.

"Nothing special in *my* bag," Kim said. And that wasn't a lie. "Besides, our class is giving everything to Children's Hospital."

"I know. And that's great," Mom told her. "It s a big help to Leslie too."

"Sure," Kim said, "on account of her diabetes."

Mom smiled and straightened the big polka dot collar on my clown costume. I knew she was telling me she was proud that I took care of my diabetes so well.

But that wasn't my problem now. It was that diamond bracelet.

I thought I had the answer the next morning when I was taking out the garbage. Mrs. Nelson, the neighbor who had the baby, was standing near her garbage can, too, only she wasn't putting garbage in. She was taking it out.

"Lose something?" I asked.

"I think little Gerri threw something valuable away."

So Kim had been right. I walked over and started to explain that I had the "something valuable." Suddenly Mrs. Nelson held up a silver spoon. "I found it!" she shouted to someone inside, and went back in.

I walked back inside, too, but I wasn't shouting like she was. I still had my mystery.

Although I hadn't believed Kim about Junior Tomkin, I couldn't help looking for him when I got to school. And he wasn't there! His friend, Jose, told me, "All of a sudden Junior had to visit his grandmother. It was kind of funny, but he just took off."

I hurried to Kim's locker and whispered the news to her. "What do you think?" I asked.

"I'll tell you what I think, Leslie. I think he stole the bracelet, got panicky, and dropped it into your bag to get rid of it. Then he left town."

"Oh, Kim. It's too much like a movie," I told her.

Still, it did fit. At least, it fit until suppertime. That's when I got the next piece of the puzzle. As I was helping Mom set the table she said, "Poor Janet Samuels. She's having so much trouble with her mother, old Mrs. Dishler."

"What kind of trouble could an old lady in a wheelchair make?" I asked, slipping the dishes into place around the table.

"Well, Mrs. Dishler seems to be giving things

away. . .expensive things. They're trying to stop her, but she still finds a way to do it. Yesterday she gave a pair of silver earrings to the nurse who helps her with her exercises."

"You mean she's giving away her daughter's things?" I asked.

"No. Not her daughter's. Her own things. Everything she gave away is hers," Mom said.

"Well, she can do that, can't she?"

"Sure, but her daughter doesn't think it's right to give such expensive gifts away," Mom said, rinsing off some glasses.

I began to think that sometimes old people have the same problem as children. Other people tell them what to do. As if grown-ups know everything that's on your mind. I stopped sliding the dishes onto the table and asked as calmly as I could, "Anything else missing?"

"Yes. An expensive diamond bracelet, and she won't tell them what she did with it."

The phone rang just then and I rushed to grab it.

"Hello."

"Hello. Is this Leslie?"

"Yes."

"Don't let them make you give it back. I want you to have it," the voice on the phone whispered.

"Who is this?" I asked.

The line went dead. But I knew who it was.

I threw on my coat and called out, "Back in a minute," and ran down the street to Mrs. Dishler's house.

I was a little scared when I lifted my hand to knock on the door. I was even more nervous when her daughter answered. "Hello, Mrs. Samuels," I said in a quiet kind of voice. "Is Mrs. Dishler here?"

"She's resting. What did you want?"

"Well, I just want to talk to her."

"Come in." I stepped into the living room. She pointed to the couch and I sat down. "What's the problem?" Mrs. Samuels asked again.

"I just wonder how Mrs. Dishler is feeling," I told her. I didn't know what words were going to come out of my own mouth next.

"To tell you the truth, she's not very well," her daughter answered.

"Please, I have to talk to her for a minute." I couldn't tell Mrs. Samuels about the bracelet. After all, I didn't want to get Mrs. Dishler into more trouble.

Mrs. Samuels looked at me kind of funny, then went through a door right off the living room. I knew it was her mother's bedroom. They gave her that room so she wouldn't have to go up the stairs.

When Mrs. Samuels came back she said, "Go on in. She wants to see you. But just stay a few minutes, please. She's not very strong."

I nodded and walked back to the bedroom. Mrs. Dishler was lying in a huge bed resting on a big bunch of embroidered pillows. She looked so little and pale, and her hair was all white, but she was smiling.

"How nice of you to come, Leslie. Did you get the present?"

"Yes, Mrs. Dishler. But I can't accept it. It's just too expensive."

"I knew you'd say that. That's why I put it into your Halloween bag."

"But why did you give it to me in the first place?"

"Because we both have diabetes dear, and because I

want you to have a long and happy life."

I looked at her wheelchair in the corner.

"Yes," she said. "That disease has been rough on me. That's because I got it 35 years ago."

"What difference does that make?" I asked.

"What difference does that make?" she repeated. "Why, 35 years ago we had none of the wonderful things you have today. Would you believe we had to test our urine to know what our sugar was? Every day when I came home from school for lunch I had to test my urine. Had to heat it in a pan on the stove. And oh, how it smelled. Sometimes it spilled, too. My poor mother. My diabetes was tough on everyone."

"Gee," I said. "That sounds awful."

"And it still didn't tell us much," Mrs. Dishler went on. "Not like your blood glucose monitors today. My doctor even told me to eat fatty foods. Would you believe? We had to fry things in fat. And we didn't have all the insulins you have today. Besides, you should see how big our needles were!"

I sat down on a little chair near the bed and thought about what it must have been like when Mrs. Dishler was my age. But before I said anything, she went on. "We took only one shot a day, but we never felt good on one shot either.

"Oh yes," she sighed, "you certainly better believe it matters when you got your diabetes."

"Wow," I said. "I didn't know all that. But I still can't take your bracelet, Mrs. Dishler. My parents would never let me keep it."

"But I want you to have it."

Mrs. Dishler and I both kind of looked out the window

wondering what else to say.

Then I had an idea. "Mrs. Dishler," I said. "Could I come by tomorrow after school?"

"Of course, but what for, dear?"

"Well, I have a gift for you, too. And you have to accept my gift if you want me to accept yours."

"You don't have to pay me back for the bracelet," she said. "It's yours."

"I know. But I want to give you something."

She laughed a little laugh and her thin body shook. "Well, I guess that's only fair. What is the gift?"

"It's me. I mean I'll come by and talk to you after school. Maybe I can push your wheelchair outside when the weather is nice. Or we could just watch television together sometime," I told her.

"That would be lovely," Mrs. Dishler said, pulling herself up a little on the bed and smiling. "And now you can keep the bracelet, right?"

"Well, I still don't think my parents would let me have it," I told her. "But I'll tell you what. I'll wear it every time I'm over here with you. Deal?"

She laughed again and brought one hand out from under the covers. I grabbed it with both of mine. Her hand was so small that I held it carefully as we shook on our bargain. "Deal," I said.

She looked tired, so I said good-bye and left the bedroom. Mrs. Samuels was in the living room and I said good-bye to her too, then got out the door fast and ran home.

I had a lot to tell everyone, starting with how a diamond bracelet got into my Halloween bag.

Diabetes Camp: New Friends and Adventures

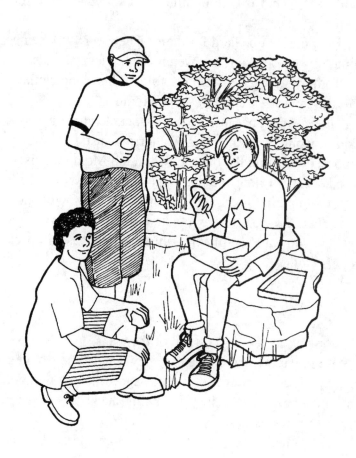

THE RED BASEBALL CAP

by Marcia Levine Mazur

Tommy was angry at his Mom and Dad. Yesterday, when he asked them whether he really had to go to diabetes camp, they only said, "You'll like it, Tommy. You'll see." They even told him, "You know, it's hard for us, too."

How could it be hard for them? They weren't leaving home for two weeks. They weren't going away alone.

Tommy watched his mother folding his camp clothes into the suitcase. He didn't say anything.

He was quiet because he had just came up with The Plan. It would work like this. Tomorrow, just when he was supposed to get on the bus, he would tell Mom that his blood sugar was low and that he felt sick. She would be afraid to put him on the bus, and it would leave without him. Then she would have to take him home again.

"Do you want the blue tee-shirt?" Mom was still packing his clothes.

"I don't care."

"I bought it just for camp."

"OK."

She put the tee-shirt on top of the jeans.

Tommy remembered the day they decided he would go to camp. It was a couple of months ago, when he first got out of the hospital. But that was before he knew how scary it was to leave home.

He had heard the night nurse tell Mom and Dad, "Everyone at the camp has diabetes. The food is terrific, and it's all the right things for kids who have diabetes.

24

There's even a full-time doctor there."

The nurse had turned to him. "You'll like it, Tommy. You'll see." She smiled. "My own son loved it."

But he wasn't her own son. Maybe her own son didn't have this scared feeling in his stomach when he thought about leaving home.

His mother stopped packing and looked at him. "Don't you feel well, Tommy?"

"I'm OK."

He wished he could just say, "I'm afraid to go. I'm afraid the camp people won't know how to take care of me. I'm afraid they won't know how much insulin I need. I'm afraid I'll get sick and have to go to the hospital."

Every morning since he came home from the hospital, Mom and Dad had helped him with his shots. And Dad watched him check his blood sugar every night. Maybe at camp he'd make a mistake.

"Mom, what if I get sick there?" Tommy couldn't forget that Sunday afternoon when he got very sick and ended up in the hospital. Mom and Dad had stayed with him the whole time.

"What if I have to go to the hospital again?" he asked while she zipped the suitcase closed.

She hugged him. "We're not far away, Tommy. And there's a doctor right there. You'll like it, Tommy. You'll see."

"Are you ready to leave for the doctor now?" she asked. They had an appointment at 11 o'clock for his camp checkup with Dr. Bloom.

"Sure," he said. But he wasn't. He didn't want to go to Dr. Bloom. He didn't want doctors or special camps. He wanted things to be like they used to be, before he got diabetes.

Neither Tommy nor his mother said anything on the

way to Dr. Bloom's.

A lot of parents and kids he knew were there. But there was one older boy he'd never seen before. He was wearing a red baseball cap, only he had it on backwards. And he was throwing a ball so high it hit the ceiling. Everyone kept looking at him. Tommy could tell they wished he would stop. As soon as Tommy walked into the waiting room, Miss Levine, the nurse, smiled at him.

"Tommy, why don't you and Junior go out and toss the ball outside?" She pointed to the boy with the backward baseball cap. "I'll let you know when Dr. Bloom is ready for you."

Tommy wasn't sure he wanted to play with Junior. He looked older and kind of mean. But Tommy only said, "Sure, Miss Levine."

Outside, Junior threw the ball before Tommy was ready. Tommy chased it and threw it back as hard as he could, but Junior caught it.

"What's your name?" Junior asked, throwing again.

"Tommy."

"That's a baby name. What's your real name?"

"Thomas."

"Mine's Junior. It's really Edward. I've got the same name as my father. I'm Edward Junior. But I didn't like it when they called me Eddie. So I told them to call me Junior. How come you're seeing Dr. Bloom, Tom?" Junior asked.

"I'm going to camp tomorrow and I have to get a checkup."

"Diabetes camp?"

"Yeah."

"I'm going in August. This is my third year. It's great.

I'll probably be a counselor when I'm older."

"I never went before."

"That's where I learned to throw." Junior threw the ball so hard Tommy dropped it.

"See?"

"Yeah."

Tommy swallowed a minute. Then he asked, "Did you ever wish your mother was there?"

"My mother? Are you kidding?" Junior threw the ball even harder. "My mother didn't even want me to go. Dr. Bloom talked her into it. Then the third day I was there I was pitching a no-hitter, and someone yelled, 'Hey, Junior, your mother's here.' I had to miss four innings to show her my cabin and everything. She thought I couldn't take care of myself."

Junior threw the ball high and Tommy jumped for it. It slapped into his hand and hurt for a minute. But Tommy didn't even feel it when Junior said, "Nice catch."

Tommy smiled.

"But weren't you scared sometimes, Junior? I mean, didn't you think something might happen?" he asked.

"Something did happen. I started to have an insulin reaction once."

Tommy forgot about throwing. "Weren't you afraid nobody would know?"

"Not at camp. You never go anywhere alone in case you have an insulin reaction. You always go with a buddy. Anyway, this one time I was throwing the ball, and I started to feel sick and my buddy ran and got Mark. He was my cabin leader."

"And what happened?" Tommy asked.

"Mark knew what to do. He's had diabetes since was

seven, just like me. He got me some sugar and told my buddy to call the nurse."

Junior threw a grounder and Tommy scooped it up. Junior kept talking.

"You know the best thing about the diabetes camp?"

"What?"

"You don't have to tell anybody you have diabetes. Everybody has it."

He added, "They go swimming, and play baseball, and tell ghost stories. You'll like it, Tom. You'll see."

Then Junior stopped throwing. He took off his red base-ball cap, and smoothed it back onto his head...backwards.

"Where did you get that cap?" Tommy asked.

"My mom bought it. I play a lot of baseball."

When Miss Levine came to the door to get Junior, he threw Tommy the ball one last time. Tommy made an easy catch. "So long, Tom. Maybe I'll teach you how to pitch next year."

Tommy was quiet when he and his mother went in to see Dr. Bloom. He barely answered the questions. But Dr. Bloom said he was in great shape. Then the doctor turned to his mother. "Don't worry. He'll be just fine." Tommy was surprised to see that his mother looked sad. He real-ized she would miss him.

Dr. Bloom turned to Tommy. "You'll like it, Tommy. You'll see," he said.

At the car, Tommy hopped in quickly. "Mom," he asked, "can I get a baseball cap?"

"That's good idea. You'll be in the sun a lot."

She stopped at a store on the way home and tried dif-ferent caps on him. But Tommy knew the one he wanted. When they left with the red cap, he smoothed it onto his head. . .backwards. He showed it to Dad that night, and he wore it the next morning when they all drove to the schoolyard where the camp bus was waiting.

When Tommy saw the big yellow bus, his stomach felt funny. There were dozens of kids there cheering and waving, dragging suitcases, carrying backpacks, calling each other's names. It was scary, but, hey, it was kind of exciting, too.

Then it was time to say good-bye. That meant it was time to work The Plan—pretending to get sick.

Mom bent down and hugged him hard. She kind of buried her face in his shirt for a minute. "Don't forget to write. We'll be thinking about you, but we know you can take care of yourself." Dad hugged him, too, very hard.

Suddenly Tommy understood something. She and Dad would miss him just as he'd miss them. Maybe they were even a little afraid to see him go. Still, no one had to talk *his* mom and dad into letting him go to camp. His mom and dad were sure he could take care of himself. That's why they were letting him go.

Instead of working The Plan, he hugged them back. "Don't worry, I'll write." He turned, took a step, then turned back and hugged Mom again. "I'll be OK. Don't worry."

And then he was on the bus, sliding into a seat next to a little boy who was waving at his mother through the window.

"What's your name?" Tommy asked him.

"Joey. What's yours?"

"Tommy," he said. "I mean Tom. How old are you?"

"Nearly seven," Joey said.

The big bus doors banged shut, the powerful motor turned over, and the bus rolled out. Joey turned in his seat so he could still see his mother as the bus moved away. Tears were rolling down his cheeks. Tommy didn't know what to say.

The bus turned the corner, and one of the counselors stood up in front. "I'm Mark," he yelled over the noise. "And I see a lot of old friends here. So I want you to get this year off with the loudest singing you can do. We're going to start with 'Row, Row, Row Your Boat.' Anybody hear of it?"

There was so much yelling, "Me!" "I did!" "Me, too!" that Mark had to put his hand up. "OK," he laughed. "You all know it. Now everybody sing."

The singing was so loud that Tommy thought the bus would lift off the ground. All the kids were almost yelling the words, "Row, row, row your boat gently down the stream. . . ."

He looked down at Joey. His little face looked white and scared. Tears were squeezing out of his eyes.

Tommy tried to call Mark to tell him the boy next to him was crying. But the singing was too loud. He looked at little Joey again. "Don't cry," he said.

But tears still rolled down his cheeks. Suddenly, Tommy took off his red baseball cap and fitted it onto Joey's head. . .backwards. Joey looked up at him, then reached out and touched the cap. He smiled at Tommy through the tears.

Tommy leaned over and yelled above the singing, "Camp will be fun, Joey. They go swimming and play baseball and tell ghost stories. And I'll teach you how to throw."

Joey looked up at him and smiled. Tommy gave him a very soft punch on the arm. "You'll like it, Joey. You'll see."

The Blue Shoe Box

By Marcia Levine Mazur

Martin sat on his bed and stared at the suitcase. He was supposed to be packing it because he was going to camp the next day. The problem was, Martin didn't want to go to camp. He didn't care that everyone said he would love it. He didn't care that all the other kids there would have diabetes just like he did. All he cared about was that it was scary going away from home alone for the first time.

"Why, you haven't even started packing!" Mom said when she saw the empty suitcase.

"Do I really have to go?" Martin asked for the fifth time.

"It will be fun," she answered him for the fifth time.

"But I won't have my rock collection with me," Martin told her. He had two rocks so far, and they meant a lot to him.

Mom stood still for a moment, then hurried out of the room, "Wait here," she called, as if he were going any-where. "I just had a great idea."

She came back with an old blue shoe box. "Why don't you pack your rock collection in this?" she asked, setting the box on the bed.

Martin picked up the box. What did he want with an old shoe box anyway? Still, he set the two rocks inside. They fit perfectly.

He lifted the pink rock and put it in the palm of his

hand. He found that if you squinted at it, it got all shimmery.

The brown rock was smaller, but a lot of thin white lines ran all through it, and that made it really neat.

Martin set the rocks back into the shoe box and put the lid on. "Wait till the kids at camp see these," he thought. Then he began packing.

By the time Mom called, "Time for your glucose check," Martin was ready.

At dinner, Dad began talking about when he went to camp. "Of course, I didn't go to a camp where all the kids had diabetes," he said.

At bedtime, Martin had his snack with Dad. He wondered if Dad had been scared the first time he went away from home, too.

Mom came in, kissed Martin goodnight, and turned off the light. "Get a good night's sleep," she said. "We want to leave by 9 tomorrow." They were going to drive him to camp.

Martin couldn't sleep, though. Questions kept going through his mind. What would it be like? What would he do there? Would he make any friends?

He yawned and turned over. Suddenly, it was morning and Mom was calling, "Hurry! The alarm clock didn't go off and we're late."

Forty-five minutes later Martin had done his glucose check, given himself his injection, had breakfast, showered, and dressed. "What a morning!" he thought as he buckled his seat belt.

"We're off!" Dad called, turning the key.

That's when Martin remembered. "Wait! I forgot my shoe box."

"Oh no," Mom groaned, but she handed him her front door key.

Martin scrambled back to his room and grabbed the shoe box. He couldn't go to camp without his rock collection!

At camp, Dad carried the suitcase into the cabin, but Martin carried the shoe box. Then Mom and Dad kissed him good-bye and drove off. Martin watched their car getting smaller as they drove away and he almost wanted to run after it.

Just then Sandy, his counselor, put his arm around Martin's shoulders and walked him inside Beech Cabin. "All our cabins are named for trees," Sandy told him.

Sandy asked the boys to tell him their names. Martin was glad that Len, Roy, and Stuart had the bunks nearest his. Then Sandy said they should give themselves a special name. "How about calling ourselves The Beech Boys?" he asked.

"Yeah," they all yelled. "We're the Beech Boys!"

Martin put his clothes in his locker but shoved his shoe box under the bed. That turned out to be a good idea, because that first night he felt a little lonely. So he just reached under his bed in the dark and pulled out his shoe box. He turned each rock over in his hand.

Suddenly Martin heard a faint sound. Someone was sniffling. It was his new friend, Len, in the bunk next to his.

"What's wrong?" Martin whispered.

"I miss my mom," Len whispered.

"Me, too," Martin answered. Then Martin had an idea. He picked up the big pink rock and handed it to Len.

"Isn't this neat?" he asked.

"Yeah." Len propped himself up on one elbow and took the rock. He lay back down still holding it in both hands. A few minutes later Martin could tell he was sleeping.

The next morning when Len said, "Here's your rock back," Martin told him, "No. You keep it."

Martin wouldn't have believed what happened next. He gave away his other rock, too!

It happened after Stuart fell and skinned his knee when the Beech Boys were on their way back from swimming. The doctor said Stuart was fine, but he couldn't go swimming for a few days.

Stuart looked so sad that Martin pulled out his shoe box and took out the brown rock.

"Here, Stuart," he said. "You can start your own rock collection while we're all swimming."

"Gee, thanks," Stuart told him.

The box was empty now, but the funny thing was, Martin felt good about it. He was glad he gave his rocks to Len and Stuart.

Then the next day at flag raising he spotted a piece of wood that looked like a bird. "Boy, look at that," he thought. He brought it back and put it in his blue shoe box.

After lunch Stuart set a rock the size of a fist on Martin's bed. It was red with black spots on one side. "Here," he said, "this is for you. It's from my new rock collection.

"Great," Martin told him, and he put the new rock into the shoe box, too. When Len saw Stuart give Martin the rock, he handed him one of his pine cones. "This is for you," he said. Len was collecting pine cones, pasting eyes and noses and ears on them. He wanted to make a whole pine cone family.

Now Martin's shoe box had more in it than when he first came. When he found a dead bug, he wrapped it in toilet paper and put that in too. Roy watched him put the bug in.

"Hey," he shouted, "I need a shoe box, for my cup." Roy had made a clay cup and painted it red.

That did it. Everyone in Beech Cabin decided he needed a shoe box, too.

Marshall, the boy whose bunk was at the far end, had made a birdhouse out of a milk carton. Charlie, who bunked right next to Marshall, was collecting leaves. Even Sandy said, "You know, I could use one of those boxes."

"I'm going to ask my mom and dad to bring me one when they pick me up," Stuart said.

"Yeah," Roy announced, "me too."

Martin felt terrific. Camp was turning out pretty neat. He didn't even think about his mom and dad much anymore. In fact, they seemed kind of far away now. All he could think about was learning to float, the play he was in—he was a clown—and the cozy feeling he had when everyone sat around the campfire at night.

His best time at camp, though, came one special night. After 'lights out,' with the moonlight shining through the window, Sandy sat in the middle of the room and began talking in a loud whisper. "This is a story about the meanest pirate who ever lived," he began, and Martin got a scary-funny feeling just waiting for the story to start.

But, there was one thing Martin didn't like about camp. Time seemed to go faster there. Mornings turned into evenings almost by magic. By the time the last day came, Martin didn't believe it was over.

On the last morning, Sandy had everyone stand in a big circle and put their arms around each other's shoulders. Then he told them to shout, "Beech Cabin is the greatest cabin ever!" It made a very loud noise. Martin couldn't remember ever feeling so happy.

Everyone exchanged names and addresses, and waited for their parents to come and take them home.

Then a funny thing happened when the parents started arriving. Every mom or dad or little sister or brother was carrying a shoe box.

Len's sister could barely see over the two she had. Stuart's mom had found a great big green one. Roy's dad handed his son a red striped box.

Slowly, the parents began looking at each other. "You brought one, too?" Len's mom said to Stuart's mom.

"What are you boys putting into those old shoe boxes?" Roy's dad asked.

Martin looked at Roy, but Roy was busy stuffing paper around his red cup and fitting it into his striped shoe box. Martin watched Stuart set his new rock collection into his green shoe box.

Len was carefully closing the lid over his pine cone family. Luckily they fitted neatly into the two shoe boxes his sister had carried in. At the other end of the cabin, Marshall had his bird feeder ready to pack, and Charlie's leaves were piled next to an extra box someone had brought.

Martin threw pine needles into his own overstuffed blue shoe box. He knew the smell of the pine needles would always remind him of Beech Cabin.

"What in the world are you boys taking home in those old boxes?" Roy's dad asked again.

Martin looked up and smiled. "I guess we're taking camp home," he said.

Growing Up:
Taking Charge

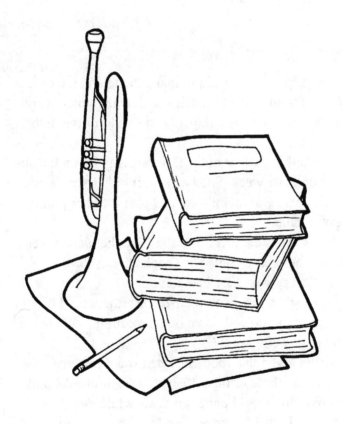

What's a Grandparent For, Anyway?

By Marcia Levine Mazur

Bertha Ross was afraid to make the telephone call. Even though it was a call she'd made hundreds of times before, today her fingers just wouldn't touch the right numbers.

All the fuss was about a Thanksgiving invitation she had mailed last week. She had sent it to her son Jerry and his wife Jean. But mainly she had sent it to her granddaughter, Diane.

It was the same invitation she gave them every year. "Would you please come for Thanksgiving?"

And every year they had come.

On the day they were to arrive, Bertha would listen for Diane jumping up and down outside calling, "We're here, Gran Gran, we're here!"

Bertha loved that moment when she threw open the door and the three of them rushed in, their cheeks pink with cold. She would unbutton coats while everyone laughed and talked at once, "Hello! How was the trip?"

But there'd be no throwing open the door this year. Bertha knew the answer to her invitation would be, "No. We're not coming."

She put down the phone and glanced around her yellow kitchen. Bertha still lived in the old house where her son Jerry grew up, and she still cooked in the kitchen where she and her late husband Daniel had enjoyed so many meals.

Right now she could almost smell the roast turkey she'd made here last Thanksgiving. How lively it had been then! Diane had been darting around the place in her bright red sweater and blue jeans, folding paper napkins, setting the table, even telling Bertha to hurry!

And that was one of Bertha's best Thanksgivings ever. What a wonderful difference it made to have the family here. If only they would come this year.

Her husband Daniel had died just after their son Jerry had married and moved away. Bertha had been so lonely after that . . . until Diane was born.

The minute Bertha Ross had picked up the soft pink blanket that held Diane, she knew there was no one else she loved the way she loved her grandchild.

She began sending her gifts. First came the soft white crib blanket Bertha knitted herself. Then there was a cloth book about Peter Rabbit followed by a red plastic train engine that whistled.

When Diane was two years old, Bertha sent her a fuzzy blue bear. Diane named it Gran Gran Bear, because her Gran Gran Bertha had sent it to her.

As the years passed, the gifts changed. There was a jump rope, a baseball, roller skates, and a pirate costume for Halloween. Sometimes Bertha whipped up a batch of cupcakes and sent them off for everyone.

Jerry would say, "You're spoiling her," and Bertha would laugh, "Well, what's a grandmother for, anyway?"

When Diane was older, she and Bertha baked chocolate chip cookies together. Once they stirred up a birthday cake for Jerry, and Bertha showed Diane how to write, "Happy Birthday, Dad," in yellow frosting.

But best of all were those holidays when Jerry and Jean and Diane rushed into the house, hugging Bertha before they had taken off their coats.

Then, suddenly—last March—everything had changed.

It began simply. Jean told Bertha that little Diane was feeling tired, that she was losing weight, and that she was drinking a lot of water and soda.

Bertha called often after that to see if Diane was better. But she wasn't. Then one evening when Bertha called about seven o'clock, there was no answer. She called and called every hour until after midnight. There was still no answer.

It was one of the worst nights of her life. She tossed and turned in bed. She sat up, switched on the bed lamp, and read for an hour. But in the morning Bertha had to laugh at herself because she couldn't remember a thing she read.

She waited for a telephone call. It was clear that Jerry and Jean were busy taking care of whatever was wrong. She didn't want to bother them; she knew it had something to do with Diane.

Finally, Jerry called. But he sounded so tired Bertha didn't mention how worried she'd been. She simply listened while he told her that they had been at the hospital all night. Diane had something called diabetes.

Bertha had sat down at her kitchen table and cried. Her little Diane in the hospital! And she was so far away. How she wanted to see them all, to hold her grandchild—just for a minute.

40

After Diane came home from the hospital, her calls were filled with words Bertha had never heard. She'd say, "Gran Gran, I have to check my blood now, and take my insulin and follow a meal plan. And I have to show my teacher how to help me if I have an insulin reaction."

Bertha began to feel left out, like she wasn't part of the family anymore.

But Bertha was pleased to see Diane acting so grown-up, taking good care of her diabetes herself.

Usually Bertha went to the movies or played cards in the evening with her friend, Shirley. Shirley always had an answer for everything. She told Bertha, "Just go and visit them. Don't ask if you can come." But Bertha didn't feel comfortable doing that.

Instead, she called. "Jerry, I'd like to come to see all of you." But Jerry didn't give her the answer she wanted. He only told her, "Maybe later, Mom. We're too busy for a visit now."

A visit! She was his mother and Jean's mother-in-law. And she was Diane's Gran Gran. She didn't want to visit. She wanted to help. She banged her hand hard against the kitchen table. Why did this darn diabetes have to come?

But Bertha didn't ask to help again.

The truth was, Bertha was afraid to offer help. Deep inside she thought they were right. What good could she be? She didn't know anything about diabetes. She couldn't even spend the afternoon alone with Diane. She didn't know what to do if something happened.

Then slowly something else began to bother her. Maybe it was all her fault. What about all those cupcakes and cookies she sent? Were they the reason Diane had diabetes?

Bertha mentioned it to Shirley, who laughed, "Don't be silly."

Still Bertha worried. And she wondered whether she and Diane would ever just cuddle up in the big chair and watch television the way they used to.

Bertha looked around her kitchen now. Maybe she'd just sell the old house. What was the point of staying here if there wouldn't be grandchildren around? She switched off the light and walked through the dark into the living room.

Suddenly, the telephone rang. She rushed back to the kitchen and grabbed the receiver.

"Hello, Jerry?"

"No. It's Shirley. Did you want to go to the movies tonight?"

"No. I'm just going to bed early."

"But I thought you were getting ready for Thanksgiving."

"There is no Thanksgiving."

"No Thanksgiving? What are you talking about?"

"I know they're not coming.

"Why ever not?"

"I told you. Because I don't know how to cook for people with diabetes."

"Well, find out."

"What?"

"Find out how to cook for someone with diabetes. I bet it's not hard."

"But I've been cooking the same way for years. How could I change?"

"You are going to have to change," Shirley said. "That little girl needs you.

"It probably wouldn't even matter if I did. They wouldn't come anyway."

"You don't know that, Bertha."

"I'm too old to learn new recipes. Goodnight, Shirl." Bertha hung up, turned off the kitchen light, and started up the stairs to her bedroom.

Then Bertha Ross did something she had never done in all the years she'd lived in her house. She stopped, turned, and sat down right on the steps.

She put her head in her hands and thought about what Shirley had said.

"Find out how to cook for someone with diabetes." Were there places you could learn about diabetes?"

It was cold and rainy the next morning, and Bertha shivered when she slipped out from under the covers. But she put on her long-sleeved blue dress, pulled her warm white sweater around her shoulders and called Shirley.

"Shirl, get ready. We're going out."

"I'm not even dressed."

"I'll be there in five minutes, so get out of bed. We're going to the library to look for books and magazines about diabetes. Maybe they have classes somewhere, too. And I'll talk to someone at the hospital if I have to."

"Hold on. I'm coming!"

A few weeks later Bertha stood in her yellow kitchen with the telephone in her hand, ready to make her call again. This time Shirley was at the table smiling at her. Bertha was still nervous about the call, but things weren't the same anymore. Today she wasn't asking for something. Today she had something to tell everyone.

Shirley gave her a thumbs up sign, and Bertha's fingers found the right numbers.

She thought about the American Diabetes Association classes she was taking and about the books and magazines the librarian had given her.

She glanced at the cookbooks waiting on the table. They had easy recipes she could hardly believe, and something called exchanges. Now, she knew that she could make a lot of foods that were on Diane's meal plan, and they were good for everyone else too. What's more, they tasted wonderful.

While the telephone rang, Bertha went over some of the new words she'd learned, like insulin, blood glucose checking, meal plans, and low blood sugar.

She even knew now that the chocolate chip cookies and cupcakes she had sent had nothing to do with Diane's diabetes. No one gets diabetes from eating sweets. Better yet, she knew that she and Diane could still cook together, as long as they made healthy things that were good for both of them.

Finally, Jean answered the phone.

"Jean, how are you? Listen, I want you and Jerry and Diane to come here for Thanksgiving. And this summer you can let Diane visit me by herself, because I have been learning all about diabetes."

Bertha put her hand over the receiver and winked at Shirley. "I don't think she believed me. She's putting Jerry on the phone."

"Jerry? You won't recognize your Mom. I'm taking classes about diabetes, and reading books and magazines. I'm going to make the best and healthiest Thanksgiving dinner you ever had."

She gave Shirley a nod. "Yes. They're coming!"

After she hung up, the two of them wrote a shopping

list. "This is going to be one great meal!" Bertha shouted out to the yellow kitchen. Then Shirley and Bertha both laughed out loud.

Finally, the Wednesday before Thanksgiving, Bertha heard Diane outside the front door calling to her again. "Gran Gran, we're here!"

Bertha yanked the door wide, letting the chilly breeze swirl in. Diane was hugging her Gran Gran Bertha even before Jerry or Jean could get inside the door.

"Mom," Jerry said, after he caught his breath, "I can't believe you took all those classes and everything."

"Of course I have." Bertha answered, "After all, what's a grandparent for, anyway?"

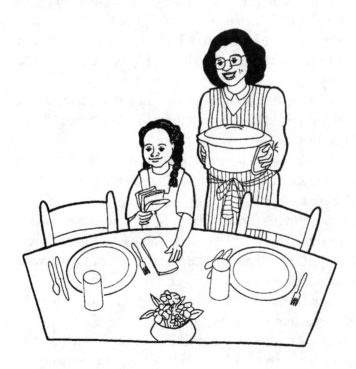

The Birthday Ghost

by Marcia Levine Mazur

L aura raced out of school the minute the last bell rang, and 17 minutes later, she was slamming her back door and darting into the kitchen.

Usually she called out, "I'm home, Mom." Today she just ran to the tray on the kitchen table and thumbed through the mail. She didn't really have to look, though. She knew the pink envelope wouldn't be there.

Everyone else's invitation had come days ago. Alison's had arrived on Monday. Sarah's and Rebecca's had come Tuesday.

Each time one of them asked Laura if she had hers yet, Laura had forced herself to sound cheerful. "Oh, it'll probably be there today."

But today was Thursday. The party was Saturday afternoon, and Laura was sure now. She wasn't going to Nora's 12th birthday party.

It wasn't fair. Sarah, Alison, Nora, and Rebecca ate lunch with Laura every day. They all went to the movies and played basketball together. But only she, Laura, was left out of the party.

When Laura looked up from the mail tray, she saw her mother watching her. "No invitation, honey?"

Laura shook her head, trying to smile. But it was hard to smile when she felt like a ball of tears was growing inside her chest.

"It's never going to come, Mom. I know. Not today, not tomorrow, not ever. And I know why."

"Maybe you should ask Nora what happened."

"I know what happened. Her mother told her not to invite me."

"But you're her friend."

"Yes, but her mother thinks I'll spoil the party because I have diabetes."

"Are you sure?"

"Oh, I'm positive. I see the way her mother looks at me when I'm over there. She thinks I eat weird food and that she'll have to watch me all the time because I'll get sick or something. So she told Nora she couldn't have me. I know."

Laura slouched into the family room and plopped down on the couch as if she'd never get up again. She hoped her mother wouldn't say something like "Well, it's not the end of the world," or, "You'll get over it."

But her mother didn't say anything at all for about five minutes. And when she did talk, she said something worse.

"I'll call Nora's mother."

"No, Mom. No. Absolutely not!"

"All right. All right. I won't call if you don't want me to. But just because you have diabetes is no reason to leave you out of a birthday party! "

Laura shrugged. "Nora's mother just doesn't understand diabetes."

Her own mother bent down and hugged her. "Now, get up and wash your face. You'll feel better." Laura walked into the bathroom as slowly as if she had nowhere else to go because that was how she felt.

The next day—Friday—was tough. Laura got through it by staying away from everyone. She even ate lunch by herself.

When the last bell rang, she charged out of school so she wouldn't see her friends. Besides, she thought, there was one last chance. Maybe the invitation had come today. She ran home, burst into the house, and went through the mail. No pink envelope.

Saturday morning dawned chilly. Mom offered to help with her morning injection. Then Dad cracked jokes all through breakfast. But she didn't feel like laughing. She knew they felt sorry for her. Getting dressed was rough too. For some reason, nothing looked good on her anymore, not even her red plaid skirt.

At lunch she pretended everything was fine so everyone would leave her alone. But everything wasn't fine. It wasn't fine at all.

"I'm going to the library," she announced, and went quickly out the door.

It was a quiet kind of day. No one was around, and the streets were empty. She wandered up one and down another, kicking the dead leaves, trying not to think. But thoughts came anyway. Why should *she* have diabetes? Why couldn't she be like everyone else?

By the time she got to the library, she was chilled and glad to bundle into the warm building. She forced herself to flip through some magazines and look at an article called, "How to Have A Great Personality."

But nothing helped. All Laura could see were her friends in their pretty blue and yellow and pink dresses, playing games, opening gifts, eating cake, and singing "Happy Birthday." She wanted to put her head on the library table and cry. She felt so alone. She looked at the library clock just at five. The birthday party was over.

Sunday came in rainy and cold. Laura thought it matched the way she felt. But she had a new problem now. What should she do at school Monday? How could she act like everything was OK? What could she say to her friends?

Strangely, that part worked out fine. It was if they had all decided that nobody would mention the party. They just stuck to subjects like homework, and how cute Jimmy was, and if Josh really liked Stacey—all the usual stuff.

Only, it wasn't usual. Laura thought they were trying too hard, talking too much. And even though no one mentioned the party, it seemed to sit on the lunchroom table like a ghost.

In fact, every time they got together after that, the ghost of Nora's party was always there.

One week passed, then another. Nora seemed to sit next to Laura more often, and Laura realized Nora wanted to make up. But Laura wasn't thinking of making up. In fact, she was wondering whether she should ever talk to any of them again. But then she'd be alone. That wasn't any good either.

Because she wasn't sure what to do, she just kept eating lunch and going to the movies with her friends, as if nothing had happened. But the ghost of Nora's party was always there with them.

Then, three weeks later, Laura's mother reminded her of something she was trying to forget. "Your birthday is two weeks off, Laura. How do you want to celebrate?"

Laura usually loved her birthday, but this year it was just another problem.

"Would you like to have your friends over?" her mother asked.

"Never," Laura whispered. "Not in a million years."

Then she started to cry. When her mother put her arms around her, Laura was surprised at how much it still hurt. It seemed like the birthday ghost lived with her even when she was alone, and she didn't know how to get rid of it.

"We'll just have a family party, then," Mom said. "You can have Grandma and Grandpa, and Uncle Len and Aunt Sarah, and they'll bring Irma and Ed, and maybe Aunt Esther will bring Norm, OK?"

"Sure. That'll be great," Laura answered softly.

But Laura knew it wouldn't be great. Family was nice, but she wanted a real party, with friends in bright dresses carrying pretty packages tied with shiny ribbons, whispering, laughing at secret jokes only they knew, because only they knew how special it was to turn 12.

That night, as she lay in bed, Laura thought about how hard it was to grow up. Why did everyone else seem to know what to do? Should she invite her friends or tell them she never wanted to see them again? How did grown-ups learn the answers?

In the dark room, she pulled the covers over her head and said, "No. I'll never invite them to my house. Never." But that only made her feel worse.

The next day her mother bought yellow paper plates with pink flowers and yellow plastic spoons and forks. She showed Laura a cake recipe that would let her stay on her meal plan.

"This is going to be a real party!" Dad laughed when he carried the bags in from the car.

But afterwards Laura knew he was wrong. It was

almost a real party. It had pink paper streamers, yellow balloons, and a "Happy Birthday" cake with yellow candles. The guests brought gifts and Laura played some of her new games with her cousins. But she knew it hadn't been a real party, not the kind of party Nora had, with all her friends around her.

Monday morning Mom packed Laura's lunch, and when Laura opened it in the lunchroom, there was a piece of birthday cake. You could still see the "Hap"on it.

"What's that?" Alison said.

"Cake."

"I thought you couldn't eat cake," Nora said.

"Sure I can eat cake, if I'm careful."

"Hey, look at that. It's a birthday cake!" Rebecca spotted the writing.

"Yesterday was my party."

The girls looked at each other as if Laura had told them she had green hair.

"Your birthday party?" Sarah repeated.

"Don't you think I can have a birthday party?"

Everyone was quiet. The ghost of Nora's party sat in the middle of the table, reminding them how they had left her out of their party.

Suddenly, Sarah reached out and plopped a piece of cake into her mouth. Alison and Rebecca broke off smaller pieces, and Nora grabbed some crumbs.

"Wow! I didn't think your cake would taste like this," Sarah told her.

"Why?' Cause I have diabetes?"

Sarah didn't answer.

"Well, there's a lot you don't know about diabetes and maybe about other things too." Laura stood up. "Maybe you don't know what it feels like to be careful what you eat all the time, or take insulin and do blood checks every day, or be left out of parties." She hadn't meant to say that last part, but once it came out, she was glad.

No one spoke. It was as if Laura had talked in some strange language they couldn't understand.

But Laura understood. She understood that her friends didn't know what to say or do any more than she did. She understood that it wasn't any easier for them to grow up than it was for her.

She looked at Nora. Nora didn't know how to tell her mother, "Laura is my friend, and I want her at my party."

And Sarah didn't know how to say, "I thought your cake wouldn't taste good because you have diabetes, but I was wrong."

And none of them knew how to tell her, "I'm sorry you weren't at the party; You should have been invited and we missed you."

Laura understood something else, too. Having diabetes, learning to take care of herself, even feeling left out sometimes, had made her a little older and—yes—a little smarter about some things.

Slowly she packed her cake back into the lunch bag. "You want to come over after school to finish my birthday cake?" she asked.

"Like we used to?" Rebecca said.

"Sure. Why not?"

The girls looked at each other, then began talking all at once. It was as if they couldn't wait to talk about parties and birthday gifts and new clothes, and all the things they hadn't talked about for weeks.

Laura smiled and felt the ghost of Nora's party

blowing away.

She felt happier than she had been for weeks. She didn't talk, though. She just listened and thought about what she had just learned—that it isn't easy for anyone to grow up, that some kids do it better than others, and that she had just done a pretty good job of it herself.

The Orange Teacher

by Marcia Levine Mazur

Rosie sat at the kitchen table spitting orange seeds into a dish. Each one landed with a "ping." She wanted to see how far she could spit the seeds, so she kept moving the dish further away. In about 15 minutes she discovered that she was able to spit an orange seed over 3 feet.

She was spitting seeds because she was trying not to think about doing her homework. And she was trying not to think about her homework because she had to write "an interesting speech" and deliver it in the front of the class the next day. And she didn't know what to write about.

Besides, she was scared to talk in front of the whole class. They'd probably all laugh at her.

So she kept spitting seeds.

Her mother came in from work, pulling off her coat and letting out a big sigh. "Whew, busy day." Then she saw the dish of seeds.

"Rosie, what on earth are you doing?"

"Spitting seeds."

"Why?"

"I can't do my homework."

"What's your homework?"

"I have to write a speech."

"Well, what's wrong with writing a speech?"

"But nothing exciting ever happens to me. Besides, I can't talk in front of the whole class."

"Of course you can. Everyone else does."

"Everyone else has something exciting to say."

"Your life is just as exciting as everyone else's."

"You don't understand."

Mrs. Burke sighed. It wasn't easy talking to Rosie
lately. Nothing Mrs. Burke said to her daughter seemed
right. It seemed as if Rosie felt different about herself and
everything else, even school, ever since she learned she
had diabetes.

Her mother tried one more time, "Honey, you do
things as well as anyone else."

"No, I don't. And anyway, everyone else doesn't have
this dumb diabetes."

Mrs. Burke turned away. There was nothing she could
say. It was true. Rosie had diabetes and none of her friends
did. But she couldn't make Rosie see that diabetes didn't
make her any different than she was before.

"I know what I'll talk on," Rosie seemed to be thinking
out loud. "I'll talk on spitting seeds. I'll call it 'Seed
Spitting."

"Oh, for heaven's sake," her mother laughed. "You're
something. Come, help me with dinner."

"What are we having?"

"Sally's Hawaiian Chicken. From the green cookbook.
I think it's recipe number 20."

Rosie pulled the green spiral cookbook off the shelf
and turned to the index in back. She found the recipe
under "Chicken."

"This is a good one, Mom. I can save the Starch
Exchange from the rice and have a pita bread instead."

"Why don't you write your speech about food
exchanges?"

"Oh, Mom, I don't want the whole world to know I
have diabetes. Besides food exchanges aren't exciting."

"But everybody likes to eat."

"Please, Mom, just forget it."

"Well, I'm afraid you still have to check your glucose now."

Rosie sighed, then brought her blood glucose checking equipment and notebook from her bedroom. She checked her blood glucose while her mom watched, then gave herself an injection, and put the kit back in her room.

By the time Dad came home, the chicken was ready, and Rosie had finished setting the table.

Just as they were done eating, Rosie's friend, Jen, barged in. "Hi. Door was open."

"That's okay, Jen. We were just finishing," Mr. Burke told her. "Sit down. Have something."

"Oh, no, thanks, Mr. Burke. I don't have much time. We have to write a speech tonight."

Mr. Burke turned to his daughter, "Rosie, what's your speech on?"

Rosie rolled her eyes at Jen as if to say, "What did you start this for?" Then she looked back at her father. "I don't know."

"Well, tell me if I can help."

Rosie asked if she could be excused and her mother and father nodded at almost the same time. She and Jen ran to her room.

"What are you going to write about?" Jen asked.

"I don't know. What are you going to write about?"

"Oh, that's easy," Jen laughed. "My trip to Disneyland. My grandmother took me last year and I have pictures and a hat and a tee-shirt and everything."

"Nothing exciting ever happens to me." Rosie dropped onto the bed.

"Too bad," Jen told her, but she didn't act like it was too bad. In fact, Rosie thought Jen was kind of glad she had such a good subject as Disneyland.

"Hey, what's this?" Jen picked up Rosie's diabetes kit.

"Nothing." Rosie grabbed it from her.

"Well, excuse me! But what is that stuff anyway?"

"It's my diabetes supplies."

"Is diabetes why you were out of school those two weeks last term?"

"If you must know, yes."

"Well, why didn't you tell us about it? All the kids were wondering."

"It's no one's business."

"But why not?"

Rosie couldn't think of an answer. How could she explain that she hadn't told her friends because she was sure they would think she was different, or that something was wrong with her? She just wanted to be the same as she always was, the same as everyone else.

"So what's diabetes anyway?" Jen was asking. "And when is it over? I mean I had the measles for two weeks, but then it went away."

"Diabetes is something you get when your body doesn't handle food exactly right. And it never goes away. You have to give yourself injections every day, and you have to eat carefully and on time, too, all the time."

"You mean you give yourself injections?"

"Twice a day."

"But that's fantastic. I could never give myself injections," Jen was looking at Rosie like she didn't really know her.

"Sure you could if you had to," Rosie said softly.

"What else do you have to do?"

"Well, I check my blood sugar."

"Say what?"

"I check my blood sugar level and I write it in a book so the doctor can see it." Rosie showed her friend the monitoring book.

Then Rosie showed her the syringe and insulin.

Jen didn't say a word. She just shook her head. "That's really brave. I mean I don't know any other kid who does all that every day."

"Well, sometimes my mom or dad help."

Then Jen jumped up as if she just thought of something.

"Hey, Rosie, you're really lucky."

"Lucky. Are you kidding?"

"You're going to have the best speech in the whole class."

"What?"

"The speech. Just tell them what you told me. Show them how you check your blood sugar, and give injections, and all that stuff."

Rosie put the supplies back on the dresser. "I don't want the whole world to know I have diabetes."

"Rosie, I can't believe you. You do all this every day, and you don't want anyone to know? Do you think the other kids could do it? Just think of them. Sarah and Debbie and Lisa and Bob and even Rich. He knows how to kick a ball, but I bet he'd be scared to give himself an injection."

Jen smiled at Rosie.

"I think you're very brave. And smart, too."

Suddenly Jen noticed Rosie's alarm clock. "Hey, I've got to go finish my own speech." She opened the door, then glanced back at Rosie. "But, you know, I don't feel so excited about it anymore. Lots of kids have gone to

Disneyland."

Rosie walked Jen to the front door, then went slowly back to her room. She pulled out her notebook and sat there thinking. A few minutes later, she started writing her speech.

Rosie gave the speech to her class the next day. Everyone listened very carefully.

When it was over, she was proud of what she'd said, and surprised at the way the kids asked her questions afterwards. It was like she was a teacher, the way they asked her about diabetes. They seemed to think doing blood glucose checks and giving yourself insulin injections was really something special.

And, she got an "A" on the speech.

Then she put it away in case she had to give another speech next year.

Rosie's Speech to Her Class

Notes to myself: Have bottle of insulin, two oranges, and two syringes (just in case), blood glucose monitor, lancets, monitoring notebook, glass of water, glucose tablets, and cake frosting gel.

Speech:
I want to tell you about something that happened to me last term, and about the way an orange actually became my teacher.

It started when I got very thirsty and had to go to the bathroom a lot. I was kind of dizzy, too. The doctor told me I had something called diabetes.

I had never heard of diabetes before. Grownups get it, too, but not the same kind kids get.

My diabetes is called insulin-dependent diabetes. That means I have to have something called insulin every day. The insulin helps my body use food. (Hold up bottle of insulin.)

You can't swallow insulin like a pill. You have to inject it. To inject myself with insulin, I use a special, very small syringe. (Hold it up.)

I learned to give myself injections by practicing on an orange, although some children learn on a doll. (Hold up orange.) I am going to show you how to inject into an orange. Then I'll let each of you try it. (Fill syringe with water from the glass. Inject into the orange. Then hand the syringe and an orange, but not the water, it's too messy) to the nearest student.

After you make an injection in the orange, please pass the syringe and the orange to the next person. While you do that, I want to tell you a little bit about diabetes.

First, there is absolutely no way you can catch it. It is not like measles or flu. It does not come from a germ or virus. Think of a sprained ankle. You can't catch that because it's not caused by a germ. And you can't catch diabetes.

Having diabetes just means that something in your body isn't handling the food you eat the way it should. And diabetes doesn't mean you can't do everything everyone else does. For instance, I am on the school soccer team, in the band, and also in the Girl Scouts.

Besides giving myself insulin shots, I also have to keep track of how much sugar I have in my blood. The sugar in your blood isn't like the sugar you put on your cereal. The sugar in your blood is called glucose, and it is made from the food you eat. To make sure my blood sugar levels are okay, I use this blood glucose monitor. (Hold up the monitor.)

I check my blood glucose two times a day, more if I don't feel well or am doing something different, like going on a trip or exercising hard. This is how I monitor my blood glucose. (Do a check. Tell the class what you are doing.)

After I'm done checking, I write down my blood glucose levels in my notebook so I can show it to the doctor. (Hold up notebook.)

When you have diabetes, it means your body has trouble handling the foods you eat. So, I have to eat carefully. But I don't have to eat special foods. The good thing is that the foods I am supposed to eat are the same foods everybody is supposed to eat, like fruits and vegetables. And junk foods for me are junk foods for everyone, like potato chips and candy. The funny thing is, people with diabetes usually eat healthier than most other people.

There is one special thing about diabetes you might need to help me with sometime. If I have too much insulin for some reason, I get something called an insulin reaction. That means my blood sugar drops too low. When that happens, I have to eat something with sugar in it right away. So I carry glucose tablets or a tube of cake frosting gel all the time, just in case I have an insulin reaction. (Hold up tablets and tube of gel.)

I can't always tell when an insulin reaction is coming

on. But if I start sweating a lot, and talking loud and kind of fast or funny, and maybe seem a little dizzy, I am probably having a reaction.

If you see me like that, please take me to the nurse or a teacher right away. If there is no one you can take me to, reach into my pocket and give me some of my cake frosting gel or a glucose tablet. Or give me orange juice, milk, or something with sugar in it, like a regular (not a diet) soda. Only give it to me if I am standing or sitting up and can drink it.

Make sure I eat or drink it, even if I say I don't need it. If I am not able to eat or drink anything, get a teacher or nurse or some other grown-up right away.

The last thing I want to tell you about diabetes is that I am going to have it all my life. But scientists are looking for a cure, so maybe one day I will be able to get rid of it.

I hope I have helped you understand about this disease. Would you like to ask me any questions?

(Note to the reader: Please do not use your lancet to check anyone else's blood glucose. Other diseases can be passed from person to person in drops of blood.)

Where is Sarah?

by Marcia Levine Mazur

It was nearly 4:30 P.M. on the day before Thanksgiving, and Sarah Davis wasn't home from school. Her father came in the door calling her, but there was no answer. That was unusual. Sarah was always waiting when her dad opened the door.

Tonight, though, no one came running out when he called.

He went into the kitchen. His wife was sitting at the table.

"Where's Sarah?" he asked.

"I don't know. She should have been here an hour ago."

"Didn't she phone?"

"No."

Mr. Davis looked out the window. Snow was starting to fall. It wasn't at all like Sarah to be late. In fact, she was the one who kept the rest of the family on time. It was Sarah who woke everyone up in the morning, calling down the hall, "Mom, Dad, you have 77 minutes to get ready." Mr. Davis called Sarah the little timekeeper.

He sat down at the table with his wife. He was worried. Besides being late, there had been other things that seemed different about Sarah lately. For one thing, she was so quiet.

Usually, Sarah was talking. Because she had diabetes, she was learning a lot about food and exercise. She was always telling them things like "You two shouldn't eat so much fat," and "Didn't you ever hear about cholesterol?"

and "Why don't you take a walk together after dinner?"

This week, though, Sarah had barely said a word at dinner. When Mr. Davis asked her what was wrong, Sarah had just said, "I'm figuring out something."

Mr. Davis thought he knew what she was figuring out.

"It's the party," he said to his wife.

She nodded. "That's what I think, too. I'll bet she was upset because there would be all those foods."

Sarah's class was having a Thanksgiving party today. There would be lots of cakes and cookies—but Sarah had been taught to be careful about what she ate.

"I offered to bake those special cookies she likes," Mrs. Davis said. "I told her she could share with her friends. But she said no."

"She's probably upset about feeling different and she's taking her time walking home," Mr. Davis answered.

"Do you think so?"

"Sure."

But neither of them was sure. It had started to snow harder and it was getting dark already. Where was Sarah?

By 4:50, Mrs. Davis started to call Sarah's friends. Yes, she had been at the party today. Yes, she had left school with everyone else.

By 5:00, Mr. Davis was ready to go out looking for her.

But just as he was starting to get his coat on, Sarah burst through the front door.

"Oh, wow, it's really cold out there," she said. There were snowflakes on the shoulders of her red coat and she was carrying an armload of books. "Mom, Dad, I'm really sorry that I'm late. It will never happen again. I promise."

"Sarah, we're not angry, but we were so worried. I was getting ready to look for you," Mr. Davis said.

Her mother bent down and took the books from Sarah. "If anything happened to you . . . "

"I knooooow, Mom," Sarah said, rolling her eyes. "You wouldn't know what to do."

Mrs. Davis pulled back a little. She looked hurt. "Sarah, we care about you."

Sarah sighed. "I know, Mom. I'm sorry I said that. And I'm sorry if I spoiled dinner. I was at the library trying to figure something out and I didn't even look at the clock."

"It must be something serious if the little timekeeper forgot to look at the clock," Mr. Davis said. "Why don't you tell us what's been bothering you.

Sarah took a deep breath. "I will," she said. "But I need to do a blood check and take my insulin. I'm getting hungry."

Sarah did her blood glucose check in the kitchen, while Mr. and Mrs. Davis got dinner ready. Half an hour later, they all sat down at the table. Mr. and Mrs. Davis had steak, French fries, and buttered peas. Sarah had a chicken breast, rice, and a salad. No one talked during dinner. Everybody seemed too nervous.

Finally, when they were done, Mr. Davis said, "Well, Sarah. I think your mother and I know what's got you so upset."

"You do?"

"Yes. We know how hard it is to be around your friends when everyone's eating cakes and cookies."

Sarah stared at her mother, then her father.

"The party, we mean," Mr. Davis said. "We know how the party upset you."

"The party was great," Sarah said.

"But weren't all the kids eating sugary things?" Mrs.

Davis said. "Sarah, I hope you watched yourself. You know, if anything hap . . ." Mrs. Davis stopped herself

"You don't have to worry, Mom," Sarah said. "When Mrs. Handy was planning the party, I went right up to her and said, 'Mrs. Handy, I don't think it's good for kids to eat so many sweets, even if they don't have diabetes. There are lots of good desserts you can make that don't have so much sugar and fat, and they're a lot better for everyone.'"

Mr. Davis laughed. "You said all that, Sarah?"

She nodded. "Yup. I gave Mrs. Handy some of the recipes Mom uses, and Mrs. Hardy did the baking. And you know what? Nobody even knew they were eating diabetic food."

"But Sarah, if everything went so well today, why have you been upset?" Mrs. Davis said.

Sarah looked down at the table.

"Sarah," her mother said again, slowly.

"I was afraid to tell you," Sarah said. "I'm worried about tomorrow.

"Tomorrow?" her mother looked surprised. "It's just Aunt Lucy and Uncle John coming for dinner. You like them."

"It's not them," Sarah said. "It's—well—it's dinner."

"But we always make you something special," Mr. Davis said. "Even a dessert."

"I know, I know," Sarah said. "But can't you see: I don't want to be special. People always ask me why I'm taking injections or why I'm doing a blood check. But I just want to be the same as everyone else. And today, at the party, I was. We all ate the same food, and nobody said, 'Sarah, what are you eating?'"

"So you would like it better if we could all have the

same thing tomorrow," Mr. Davis said.

Sarah looked at him. "Not just tomorrow, Dad. Every day. I mean, chicken and rice and lots of vegetables would be better for you and Mom, too. I know you say you're a meat and potatoes man, but there are other meats and potatoes besides steak and French fries."

Mr. Davis laughed. "I suppose there are, Sarah."

Sarah went on. "And tomorrow, you know, Aunt Lucy and Uncle John shouldn't stuff themselves. They both weigh about 800 pounds, anyway."

"Sarah!" Mrs. Davis said. But she couldn't help laughing.

"I wonder how we could make a Thanksgiving dinner that would be good for Sarah and everyone?" Mrs. Davis said.

"That's what I've been figuring out," Sarah said. She got up, ran to the hallway, and got the books she had brought home. When she came back she put them on the table. They were all cookbooks. "See, I found all of these neat recipes."

Mr. and Mrs. Davis thumbed through the cookbooks. "I guess even a meat and fries man could eat some of this," Mr. Davis said.

Sarah bit her lip. "I hope you're not angry with me. It's just that I feel I'm always a problem, the way you have to make special things for me. I don't want to be your problem. I want to be your daughter."

"Oh, Sarah," Mrs. Davis said, and gave Sarah a big hug. "I don't know why I ever worry about you. You're always going to watch your health."

Sarah smiled and said, "I want you to watch your health, too."

Sleepy Summer

By Marcia Levine Mazur

K evin woke up and saw the sun shining through the blue bedroom curtains. Two robins were singing away just outside his window.

He stretched his legs under the soft quilt. He'd sleep 15 more minutes, then maybe go bike riding with Neil. Next week, he would be leaving for diabetes camp. What a great summer this was, one of the best he could remember.

And it had started out as the worst.

He remembered the day he and Mom sat in Dr. Shapiro's office. Even now, he could almost hear the doctor ask him, "How are you feeling, Kevin?"

"OK."

"He's doing wonderfully, doctor," Kevin's mother had added. "We're so proud of him."

"How's school, Kevin?" the doctor had asked.

"OK."

"He's going to be on the honor roll again, Doctor. And he's trying out for school band," Mrs. Morris said.

"That's fine," Dr. Shapiro said, looking at Kevin, "as long as you can handle it." He stood up. "We'll have your tests in a few days, and I'll call if there's anything to discuss."

While Mrs. Morris stopped to say good-bye to the nurse, Kevin walked straight out to the car.

Mrs. Morris came out quickly. "Ill get you back to school in time for music, Kev," she told him, turning the key. "Don't worry. I know how much you want to make the band."

Kevin was quiet all the way to school. When they got there, he just opened the door and ran off. "Bye, Mom."

Just when he was at the school door, his mother called, "Kevin! You forgot your trumpet."

Kevin turned and walked back. Mrs. Morris handed the black case through the window. "You feel ok, Kevin?"

"Sure, Mom."

Kevin ran back to the school. He knew his mother was watching him.

As he rushed toward the band room, he heard the usual screeching noises. Mr. King had everyone practicing different instruments. Usually, Kevin thought the noises were pretty funny, and he and his friend Neil laughed at them. But he didn't even smile today.

Mr. King saw him come in. "You're late, Kevin."

"I was at the doctor."

"Oh, yes. I saw your note. Come in my office a minute, please."

Kevin walked through the noisy room into Mr. King's small office in back. It smelled like the old leather instrument cases he kept there.

He knew Mr. King was going to talk to him soon, but he thought it might be next week, when report cards were due.

"Kevin, you know you don't seem to be practicing the way I expected."

"I know."

"What seems to be the matter?"

"I don't know. I guess I have so much to do every night."

"What do you have to do?"

"Well, I'm trying to make the honor roll like last year, but I have Miss Herbert for history, and she gives a lot of homework. And I have the special English class with Miss Brelsford, and she gives a lot of homework, too."

"Maybe the honor roll isn't possible this time, Kevin. And I don't think your heart is in your music. Have you told your parents you're having a tough year?"

"They'd be disappointed in me."

"Well, Kevin, it's up to you. But I'm afraid you won't be making the band."

"I know. Can I go now?"

"Sure. I'll see you tomorrow."

Kevin felt like crying. He could barely walk out without the tears coming, and he almost ran from Mr. King's office and the funny noises. He forgot his trumpet again.

It was the first thing his mother remembered when she came in that evening. "Why aren't you practicing?"

"I left my trumpet at school."

"Oh, Kevin, why can't you remember things?"

"I don't know."

"Well, do your blood check and take your insulin. We'll get ready to eat."

"Will you watch me, Mom?"

"You're a smart boy, Kevin. You can take care of your diabetes by yourself."

Kevin went upstairs, but he didn't do his blood test. He lay on his bed. He felt worried, but he couldn't sleep.

How was he going to tell Mom and Dad he didn't make the band? How was he going to bring home that disappointing report card next week?

He heard Mom calling. "Remember your injection, Kevin."

It seemed to Kevin there was always something to remember. Do his blood check, take his injection, get washed, comb his hair, study, help with the dishes, do his homework, practice his music, eat his snack. He was even supposed to ride his bike at least a half an hour a day.

Mom worked until 5, and Dad got home a little later. He felt good because they trusted him to do everything himself, but sometimes it was really tough. Mom always called up late in the afternoon to see how he was doing. She'd remind him to do his blood check, and she always told him how proud they were.

He had even heard Mom or Dad tell other people how good his grades were, or how well he handled his diabetes.

How could he tell them he wasn't always sure he had done his blood check right? How could he tell them some days he didn't check at all? How could he say he wasn't always as perfect as they thought he was?

He washed his hands, took his injection, and came downstairs.

"I'm making your favorite, Kevin—spaghetti," Mom said.

Kevin tried to smile, but he really wanted to tell her that he wasn't going to be on the honor roll this year. When Dad came home and asked how the doctor's visit went, Kevin just said, "OK."

"That's my boy," Dad said.

Kevin walked out of the room. It didn't make sense. He'd be sitting down to eat with Mom and Dad in a minute, but he still felt so lonely.

The next week was awful. Report cards were due Friday, and one by one his teachers called him in and told him he wasn't doing as well as last year.

"What's wrong?" Miss Herbert asked.

"I don't know," he said. "It was just a lot harder this year."

Finally, it was Friday, report card day. His grades were as low as he expected. His friend, Neil, had done a little better, but neither made the honor roll.

"I can't bring my report card home, Neil," Kevin told him. "They always think I'm so smart."

"Just because you didn't get a good report card doesn't mean you're not smart, Kev."

"I know. But they'll be disappointed."

Neil smiled, "You know how you're always forgetting everything? Just say you forgot the report card."

Kevin knew it was a joke, but nothing seemed funny to him. "No. I can't do that, Neil." He felt so unhappy.

Then something happened.

Dr. Shapiro called Mom at work and said he'd like to see Kevin. He'd make room for him at four.

Mom called the school and left a message that she would pick up Kevin.

At the doctor's office, Dr. Shapiro wanted to see Kevin alone. "Kevin," Dr. Shapiro started, "your tests show us that your diabetes needs to be in better control. That means something isn't going right. Let's find out what it is. I know some kids who come here have a tough time doing their own blood glucose checks and taking their injections every single day."

"Really?" Kevin asked.

"I also see kids who are worried about different things, so it's hard for them to stay on track with their diabetes care."

Then Kevin told Dr. Shapiro he was kind of worried, too. He told him what Mr. King had said, and about his grades, and about all the homework, and how Mom and Dad thought he would be on the honor roll. He told the doctor that he did his glucose checks and took his insulin shots by himself. Still, he didn't always feel grown-up enough to do his diabetes care on his own.

The doctor listened quietly while Kevin told him that he didn't want to disappoint Mom and Dad. They thought so much of him.

Dr. Shapiro looked at Kevin a minute before he spoke. Then he said, "Kevin, let me tell you a story. When I was your age, I wanted to be a doctor. It was all I ever wanted to be. But it cost a lot of money to go to medical school, so my parents saved money for years.

"Then I got into medical school. And the first year was harder than I expected. In fact, it was so hard I thought I'd have to quit. But I knew how much it would disappoint not only me, but my mother and father.

"So I signed up for summer school, and I took a lot of medical books out of the library. I wanted to read them all before school started again in the fall.

"You know what my mother said?"

"What?" Kevin asked He didn't really see what this had to do with him.

"My mother said, 'Not this year. This is the year for a sleepy summer.' "

"A sleepy summer?" Kevin asked.

"I could hardly believe she was saying that, because she always wanted me to study," Dr. Shapiro added. "But I did what she said. Of course, school was still hard the next year. But I felt more relaxed, and I did better.

"I found out my mother was right. Sometimes, every-one needs a little break. Sometimes it's a chance to drop a class, or stop taking music lessons for awhile, sleep late on week-ends, or let someone else take over the injections once in a while. And sometimes it's one sleepy summer."

"But my mom and dad will never understand," Kevin

told Dr. Shapiro. "Maybe you could explain to them about the sleepy summer."

"Well, I could, Kevin," Dr. Shapiro told him, "but they're your parents. You know how much you love them, and you know how much they love you.

"Besides," he added, "Sometimes, telling people how you feel is a kind of gift. But it's a gift only you can give."

The next morning Kevin pulled the quilt over his head to keep the sunshine out. He remembered all the things he had said the night before when Mom and Dad asked him about his report card.

He even remembered that he cried a little when he told them he didn't want to disappoint them.

He let them know how he still wanted them to watch him do his glucose checks and take his insulin. And he explained how tough it was to get up Saturday or Sunday mornings to take care of his diabetes.

They talked to him, too. They told him how much they loved him, and that they would always be proud of him. They said it wasn't his grades that made them proud, it was just him. And they wanted to help him whenever they could.

They said they had a lot of things on their minds, too. They hadn't realized how hard the year had been for him. They had no idea he wanted them to watch him with his diabetes care. They were happy they could give him a break once in awhile and take over the injections some mornings.

Kevin punched his pillow to fluff it up. He heard Neil outside calling.

Dr. Shapiro's mother sure was right. Sometimes everyone needs to let things go a little, to let someone else help out. Sometimes everyone just needs a sleepy summer.

A Problem Named Charlie

by Marcia Levine Mazur

Have you ever done anything dumb? I did. About a month ago. I got rid of my mother's boyfriend Charlie.

It happened like this. My mom and dad were divorced when I was a baby, so I don't remember them ever being together. I visit my dad once a month, of course, but mostly I live with my mom.

And everything was going fine until a couple of months ago. That's when my mom brought Charlie Stanford home.

At first I kind of felt sorry for Charlie. He couldn't do anything—I mean anything—right. For instance, the first thing he did when my mom introduced us was hand me a great big candy bar.

"Oh, no," Mom said real fast. "I told you Brad has diabetes. That's not what he should eat."

"Oh, come on, Dorothy, he's just a kid," Charlie said, and smiled at me.

"It's not like that. He has to watch what he eats," she told him. I could tell she was angry.

"Sorry," he told her, and put the candy bar back in his pocket. Then he just stood there.

I felt sorry for old Charlie so I asked him to go outside and play catch with me. But the first ball he threw went way over my head, and the second hit me in the knee. So I said that it was getting dark anyhow and it was time to stop playing.

That night I asked Mom if she was going to marry Charlie Stanford. She kind of combed my hair with her fingers and said, "I just might, honey. What do you think?"

"I think we don't need him," I told her. "Besides, I already have Dad."

"Well, of course, Dad will always be your father. But I'm kind of lonely. I mean I'm lonely for a grown-up in the house." She kissed me goodnight and I snuggled down into bed, but I knew I had a problem, and it's name was Charlie.

About a week later Mom invited Charlie to my school night, and he really messed up then. Right when Mr. Selhub lifted his baton and we all took a deep breath and started singing "Bless This House," Charlie began to sneeze. I mean he sneezed so much he had to leave the room! Mom stayed, of course, but everyone was giggling, and I just wished the whole thing was over.

I could go on and on about Charlie, like the time Mom asked him to pick up a sweater for her that was on sale, and he bought the wrong size and the wrong color. All the time I kept telling her, "We don't need him, Mom. He'll never work out." And I intended to make sure he didn't.

If you wonder why I wanted to get rid of Charlie, I'll tell you. He changed everything. I mean, he was always there, opening the door for her, bringing her flowers. He dropped over on Wednesday evenings after work, and he came for dinner Friday night. And of course, Mom had to make Charlie's favorite food—fish—instead of my macaroni and cheese.

But the worst was Saturday. He was there all day watering the lawn, fixing the drains, painting the porch or some darn thing. It was just like he lived there. And he and Mom were always smiling at each other.

Oh sure, he asked me about school, and he even

offered to play baseball again. I took him up on it, but after that second time I could see that Charlie Stanford would need seventeen strikes to get one hit.

It was clear that we just weren't getting along. But everything burst apart when Charlie came up with his so-called brilliant idea.

He invited me out to eat, just the two of us, to a place called the Sherwood Forest. That's this dopey restaurant where they have birds in cages and the tables are made out of logs and stuff. Afterwards, we were going to meet Mom and the three of us would go to the movies.

Of course, he invited me right in front of Mom, and she said, "What a nice invitation," so I had to say I'd go.

Sure enough, the next Friday night Charlie showed up, and when I answered the door he said something really nerdy like, "Does Mr. Brad Simons live here?"

Just as we were leaving the house I heard Mom tell Charlie to be careful about what I ate.

But that night at the restaurant old Charlie finally blew it. He reminded me of Grandma who always tells me it's OK to eat all the cake I want ,cause it's my birthday." Charlie said to me, "It's a special night, kid. Why don't you lighten up and go off the diet?"

If there's one thing that gets my Mom mad, it's people who don't understand about my diabetes. And Charlie still didn't get it. I mean, he still didn't have a clue that people with diabetes shouldn't just eat anything they want, no matter what special night it is.

At first I thought I'd get him in real trouble by order-ing a fried chop, a double order of French fries, and a big piece of chocolate cake.

But then I said to myself, "Naaah. Why should I get

sick just because Charlie doesn't understand diabetes?" So I ordered macaroni and cheese and a diet soda. I was so full I didn't have to worry about desert.

It seemed like it took forever for the food to come, and I didn't know what to talk about, so I asked Charlie if he always wore glasses. "Ever since I was three years old," he said in a kind of sad voice. "And I always hated them."

I tried to imagine "little boy Charlie," a nerdy kid who couldn't play baseball and had to wear thick glasses. That picture made me want to cheer him up, so I asked where he worked and he said, "Downtown on Calvert Street. Say, why don't you come and visit me sometime? I'd be so proud to show you around."

Then he did something no one else ever did before. He took out this neat leather case, pulled out his card, and handed it to me over the table. It had fancy black writing, and I stuck it in my shirt pocket.

"Maybe I will," I said.

I knew Charlie had tried to be nice to me, but when Mom asked me how the dinner was, I told her I ate macaroni and cheese and a diet soda, even though Charlie had said I could forget my diabetes and eat anything I wanted.

"He what?!"

That started it. They argued all through the movie, and I loved it. She said things like, "Don't you realize he could have gotten sick?" and he said, "But he's just a kid," until everyone around us started shushing them. After that they barely talked the rest of the evening.

At least until I went to bed. Then they really went at it. She said "Maybe you're not the person I thought you were."

And he said, "But I just wanted him to have a good

time."

After that Charlie didn't come around anymore, and I was really glad. Finally, things would get back to normal. Only they didn't. Mom was sad all the time, and one night I heard her crying.

So I thought about it on my way to school every day and I decided that having old Charlie around wasn't as bad as all that. In fact, he was kind of fun when you thought about it.

But mainly, I knew I was the person who had made Mom unhappy.

So one afternoon I took out Charlie's card and called him. A woman answered and when I said I wanted to speak to Mr. Stanford, she said "Oh, you're in luck. He's just come out of his meeting."

Then Charlie was on the phone. He seemed really glad to hear from me. "Is everything OK?" he asked.

"Oh, sure," I told him. "But I got this idea."

"Shoot," he said. And then I talked and talked and explained my idea, and he listened so quietly I wasn't sure he was still there. But when I was done, he was so excited he started to hang up without saying good-bye. I knew that was just Charlie, though. Anyway, he caught himself, and thanked me a hundred times.

And then I waited and waited, but nothing happened. Of course, I knew my plan would take a couple of weeks, but it was over a month already, and no one heard anything from old Charlie.

Mom didn't know I had talked to him of course, and I didn't see any need to tell her because it looked like my plan wasn't working anyway. Maybe he had just said the heck with both of us. Grown-ups can do funny things like that, you know.

Then, last Saturday, he called. Mom picked up the phone and whispered to me, "It's Charlie." A few minutes later she covered the mouthpiece and said, "He wants to come over tonight." I nodded "yes," real hard.

When Charlie came to the door he had two packages all wrapped with red ribbons. Mine was kind of big but Mom's was real small. He gave me mine first.

I ripped off the paper. He had packed four apples, three oranges, and a bunch of carrots in a box. Mom looked confused, but I laughed out loud really hard.

Then she opened hers. Inside was a little piece of paper. She unfolded it very carefully.

It was a certificate that said Charlie had passed a diabetes education course. She started to laugh and then she started to cry. She threw her arms around him, and I kind of hugged him around the middle. Then Charlie took one arm off Mom and put it around me and, to tell you the truth, it felt kind of warm and nice.

"It was Brad's idea," he told her. "He's a great kid and you're right. We have to take good care of him."

You know, I think it's going to be fun to teach Charlie to play baseball. But I think it's going to take the rest of my life to do it.

MY FAMILY AND ME

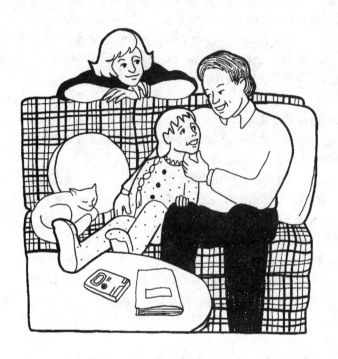

Megan's Secret

by Marcia Levine Mazur

Megan's dad had left yesterday, Friday. He and
Megan's mom had had another argument, and he
had slammed out the front door and was gone.

Now it was Saturday morning, the first Saturday in
Megan's life that she didn't want to watch a single cartoon
or even get out of bed.

She didn't want to call Buddy to see if they could race
skateboards either. And she wasn't hungry. She didn't
want any breakfast. She just wanted to pull the covers up
over her head and never get up again.

Dad had left during supper, right in the middle of yet
another argument he and her Mom were having. Usually,
Megan put her hands over her ears to block out the sound
when Mom and Dad argued. She didn't want to hear it; it
was awful.

But this time was different. This time, even after
Megan walked away she could still hear them through the
wall. Even after she shut her door, their voices came into
the room.

And this time Mom didn't run up to their bedroom crying. This time Dad left, shouting, "I've had it."

Mom had shouted back, "Go on. Get out." Then
Megan heard the front door slam, and he was gone.

An hour later, her mother had come into Megan's room
and hugged her.

"Won't I ever see Dad again?"

"Of course you will, honey. I'm sure he'll call soon."

82

Mom brought Megan's bedtime snack. The two of them sat on the side of the bed munching crackers and drinking skim milk. They even laughed out loud at the chomping sound the crackers made.

Afterwards, her mother tucked the covers under Megan's chin, kissed her, and whispered, "Everything will be OK, honey. You'll see."

But Megan didn't see. Nothing would ever be OK again.

During the night she heard Mom tiptoe in to look at her. Megan knew Mom felt bad, but she didn't want to talk, even though Megan liked the feel of Mom's hand stroking her forehead.

Still, she pretended to be asleep.

Now it was Saturday morning--but so different from last Saturday. Then Dad had called out from the living room, "Where's Megan? I can't find Megan. I want to watch her do her glucose check."

And Megan had laughed and rushed over in her pajamas carrying her glucose meter and record book. She checked her blood glucose level while Dad watched.

During the week, he and Mom took turns watching her, but everyone was always in such a hurry then.

Saturdays were different. It was always Dad's turn on Saturday. He was so funny, sometimes making jokes like the one where she might say, "Did you forget about going skating this afternoon?' and he'd say. "Me forget? I got a memory like an elephant."

Last Saturday he'd thumbed through her record note-book and slapped it onto the table. "Hey, kiddo," he announced. "It's time for a new book. What color do you want?"

"I don't know," she shrugged.

"Well, pick whatever color you want in the whole world. And if they don't have it, we'll write to the factory and tell them to make it."

She had known then that he was kidding about writing to the factory. Now she wondered if he was kidding about getting the book, too.

Mom came into her bedroom and opened the blinds, letting the sunlight rush in and brighten the whole room. "Good morning, Megan. Sleep well?"

Megan barely whispered, "Good morning." She wished Mom hadn't let the light in. She hid under the covers again, where it was warm and safe.

Mom gently tugged the covers off. "Tell you what, Megan. I'll give your injections today. And I'll even look."

Megan knew Mom was trying to be funny because that was a joke they had. The first time Mom had given Megan's injection she had said, "I don't mind doing it. I just don't want to look," and they had laughed, all three of them.

Megan looked up at her mother. "Why did he leave, Mom?"

Mrs. Mitchell sat down on the edge of the bed. "Well, sometimes things just don't work out the way you want them to, Megan. It's no one's fault."

But Megan knew better. It was someone's fault—hers. That was her secret. If she had been a better girl, if she had done her homework every night, if she had always listened to what they told her, Mom and Dad wouldn't have argued all the time. They'd have been happy.

If she had been really, really nice, Dad wouldn't have left.

She thought about those two Cs on her last report card,

and the way she wouldn't turn off the television sometime, and her room. Oh boy, her room was a mess!

But mostly, she thought about her diabetes. She was sure they wouldn't have argued so much if they didn't have to take her to the doctor all the time, and make sure she ate the right foods, and help her check her glucose and inject insulin, and watch for reactions.

Megan wanted to tell her mother that she would be good, the best girl in the whole world, and that Dad didn't have to go away.

But she didn't want her mother to know her secret, the secret of whose fault it was. So she just pulled the covers over her head and pretended she was in a little tent, and Dad would be home again when she came out of her tent.

But he wasn't there when Mom gently slipped the covers off. "Come on," she said softly, "Time to get up and get on with things. "

"I don't want to get on with things. I don't want to take any more shots. Maybe if I didn't have to take insulin then Dad wouldn't have gone away." she finally said.

"But, what do your injections have to do with Dad going away?"

Megan turned toward the wall. She was almost telling Mom the secret.

Suddenly the phone rang. Before Megan could get her feet to the floor, Mom was running faster than Megan ever saw her run before. Megan knew Mom was thinking the same thing she was. It was Dad calling. He was coming back.

But it wasn't Dad.

"Buddy wants to know if you can skateboard with him," Mom called to her.

"I don't want to."

"Go ahead, Megan. You don't want to stay in the house."

"Yes, I do."

Mom came back to the room. "Tell you what, honey. When Dad calls, I'll get his number and you can call him back. In the meantime, you get dressed and go on out with Buddy."

When Megan heard Buddy at the door, she pulled on her pink jacket, grabbed her skateboard, and ran out.

Megan always felt good in her pink jacket. Pink was really her favorite color. She'd tell Dad that.

Buddy had one foot on his skateboard, and began pushing off even while he was calling, "Hi."

"Hey, don't you even wait to say hello?" Megan shouted at him.

"Race you to the schoolyard," he called back.

Usually, Megan hopped onto her board, too, but this time she called, "You're cheating."

"Am not."

"Are too. You started first."

Buddy stopped half a block away.

"Come on, Megan."

"Why should I? You didn't even wait for me."

"Well, I'm waiting now."

"I don't want to go to the schoolyard. I want to go the other way."

"But we always go to the schoolyard," Buddy complained.

"Well, I don't want to go there now. Besides, why did you wear that yucky green sweater. You know I hate it.

"Well, I like it."

"Well, I hate it."

"Well, it's none of your business what I wear."

"Well, I have to look at it."

"Hey, Meggie, what's wrong with you anyway?"

Megan got on her board and slapped one foot on the sidewalk until she went past Buddy, but when she turned to look back at him, her board swerved and she fell. Suddenly she was lying on the chilly ground, her skateboard skidding away in front, her knee bleeding.

"Look what you made me do, Buddy Gordon!"

"Me? I didn't make you do it."

"Yes, you did."

"Anyway, you're not hurt. Come on, let's go to the schoolyard."

"I told you. I don't want to go to the dumb schoolyard."

"Well, I'm going by myself."

"Go ahead. I never want to see you again, anyway." Buddy skated over and held out his hand to help her up. Megan slapped it away, so Buddy skated off.

Megan still sat on the ground, feeling cold and alone, and suddenly she just started to cry.

She cried and cried, but no one seemed to hear. Finally, she swallowed hard, wiped her tears, and stood up again.

Carrying her board on her shoulder, she walked back into the house and found Mom sitting at the kitchen table. "What happened? Where's Buddy?"

"We had a fight. I never want to see him again."

Her mother looked at her a minute, then quietly set the skateboard on the floor. She put her hands on Megan's shoulders. "Oh, Megan, please forgive me for making you have a fight with Buddy. I'll be a better mother so you can be friends with Buddy again."

"What are you talking about? It's not your fault Buddy

and I had a fight."

"You're right. It's not. And it's not your fault that your Dad and I had one."

Megan stood still a minute, then hugged her mother very hard. She was still hugging her when the phone rang. "I think it's for you," Mom said softly.

Megan grabbed the phone. "Dad?"

"Hi, kiddo. How you doing?" It was the same laughing way he sometimes talked to her.

"Are you coming back?"

"No, honey. I'm going to be living somewhere else for awhile. But you and I have a date next Saturday afternoon. We're going to get you that record book."

"I thought you forgot."

"Me forget? I got a memory like an elephant. What color did you want?"

"Pink."

"Well, we'll get you the pinkest book in the whole world, and if it's not pink enough . . . "

"I know. We'll send it back to the factory to make it pinker."

"You got it."

"Dad, where are you?"

"I'm at a friend's house now, but I'll have a place of my own soon, and you'll come and stay with me sometimes."

"I will?"

"Of course. You know, kiddo, you should get a memory like an elephant, too. You're forgetting something important."

"I am? What?"

"That it doesn't matter where I live. I'll always be your Dad."

Grandma and Me

by Marcia Levine Mazur

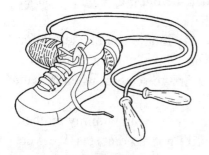

I woke up an hour early last Monday, because I was worried. About Grandma. See, I had to tell my teacher if I was coming to Parents' Night that Friday night. (Parents' Night is when we bring our parents to school so they can talk to our teachers.)

But even though I live with Grandma, I didn't want to bring her to Parents' Night. I mean, she's not really my parent, is she?

Besides, she dresses kind of funny. You should see this old black coat she wears. It must be a million years old, and she wears big white sneakers, too. I mean, they must be two sizes too big. That's because her feet hurt. And she's always saying, "I'm so tired I don't think I'll ever move again." Then she sits down in her big chair and falls asleep.

Of course, she does work hard all day. Grandma takes care of three babies so their mothers and fathers can go to work. That's how she makes her money.

Anyway, like I say, she's my Grandma, and I didn't see why I had to take her to Parents' Night. I mean, I do have a mother. I just don't live with her.

My mother's name is Ilona. Isn't that pretty? She's pretty, too. She has long dark hair and she wears red nail polish. When I lived with her she put polish on my nails, too. Grandma doesn't do that.

I never knew my father. My mother said he left before I was born, but she never said where he went. I used to watch the door so I'd be the first to see him when he came back. But he never did.

Anyway, that was when I was living with my mother, but I only lived with her until I got my diabetes. We were in a little apartment then, and my mother and I had to sleep in the same bedroom.

Then last summer I started getting sick. You know, thirsty and kind of dizzy. I remember Grandma telling my mother, "Ilona, you take her to a doctor." But when the doctor said I had diabetes, my mother started to cry—right there in his office. I didn't know what to do.

Back at the apartment, Mamma called Grandma. "I can hardly take care of this baby as it is," she told Grandma. "and now she has diabetes."

I felt like it was all my fault, and I told Mamma I would be a really good girl, and never have diabetes again. But she just kissed me on the forehead and said Grandma was coming over.

Grandma did come over, and I heard her and Mamma talking in the kitchen—pretty loud, sometimes. Then Grandma put my clothes in a suitcase, and told me I was going to live with her. I hugged my mother good-bye and she said not to worry, that she would come and visit.

So now I live with Grandma, but my mother doesn't come to visit very much. She's a waitress, you know, and she's very busy, but I do talk to her on the phone sometimes.

And that's how all the trouble started.

Like I said, last Monday I had to tell the teacher whether I'd be at Parents' Night on Friday. But I had this problem. What to do about Grandma?

So, while I was lying in bed after waking up early, I decided I would invite my mother to Parents' Night. But I didn't want to hurt Grandma's feelings. Anyway, I worked out this plan.

I would come home from school early that afternoon instead of going to Barbara's house to play. Then, when Grandma was taking care of the babies, I would go into her bedroom and call my mother on that phone next to her bed.

To make sure my plan worked, I had to pretend that today was just like any other day. So I got up, ran into Grandma's bedroom in my pajamas. checked my blood glucose with her like always, and wrote the numbers in my book. Then I sat on the bed while she gave me my insulin injection.

That's because I have diabetes, of course.

After that I got dressed and had breakfast in the kitchen while Mrs. Pinchot, Mrs. Beltzer, and Mr. Jameson dropped off their babies. That's how the mornings always are at Grandma's house.

But today was different, at least inside of me, because I knew that I wasn't telling Grandma about Parents' Night. I went to school, and came home early like I planned. But as I was walking up the porch steps, I saw Grandma sitting there with the three babies. Two were in their playpens, but little Joseph Pinchot was in her lap.

"Why are you home so early, Valerie?" she asked me.

"Oh, nothing special," I said, and picked up my jump rope from under the porch steps where I always left it.

And you know what happened then? Grandma put little Joseph in the playpen, came down the steps and held out her hand for the rope. I gave it to her. and she started jumping! She only got to seven, but I mean, Grandma jumping rope!

"Grandma, I didn't know you could jump rope," I told her.

She laughed. "I used to jump with your mother when she was your age.

Grandma went back up on the porch, kind of fanning herself with her hand. I guess the jumping made her warm. Anyway, she was waiting for the parents to come for their babies, and that worked out perfect for me.

With Grandma on the porch, I could go into her bedroom and call my mother. It took about eight rings before she answered. "Hello."

"Hello, Mamma, this is Valerie.

"Val, honey, is something wrong?"

"Oh, no. I just wanted to talk to you.

"Well, that's nice.

"I want to know if you can come to Parents' Night at school this Friday."

She was quiet a minute. "Oh, Val, honey, I don't think I can. Why don't you ask Grandma to take you?"

"But it's Parents' Night."

"I' m sorry, honey. I have the dinner shift at the restaurant. But, Val, we'll go to a movie some time soon, OK?"

"Sure, Mamma. OK. Good-bye."

"Good-bye. Say hello to Grandma."

I felt bad when I hung up the phone. But I felt a lot

worse when I looked up and saw Grandma standing in the doorway.

She turned and walked out without saying a word, and my stomach seemed to fall below my knees. I knew she heard me ask my mother to Parents' Night.

I walked back onto the porch again, but it was empty now. I could hear Mrs. Beltzer and Mr. Jameson inside picking up their babies so I started jumping rope again. But I stopped. I really didn't feel like jumping anymore.

Then Mrs. Pinchot came for little Joseph. "Hi, Valerie," she called. "Where's your grandmother?"

"Inside."

"Well, it's good to see you, Valerie. You know, I'm sure glad you came to live with your grandma."

"You are? Why?"

"Because if you hadn't moved in, she wouldn't have taken Joseph."

"What do you mean?"

"Well, she only took care of one baby until you came. But then she took on two more. I guess she needed the money.

"I didn't know that."

"Oh, she didn't tell you?" Mrs. Pinchot was already inside the house.

It seemed colder outside now, as if the sun had gone away. So I went into the house too, and sat on my bed. I didn't know Grandma had taken in more babies when I came. Just like I didn't know Grandma could jump rope.

Mostly I didn't know how bad I'd feel about hurting her, and now I didn't even want to go into the kitchen because I knew she was alone in there. Finally, I heard her calling.

"Val, honey, time to do your glucose check and get your shot."

I took my supplies from the dresser and sort of dragged into the kitchen.

Grandma was standing at the sink mashing the potatoes. Her sneakers were untied so I knew her feet hurt, but she watched me check my glucose and then she gave me my insulin injection.

Finally, I couldn't stand the quiet, so I said, "Grandma, I'm sorry I didn't tell you about Parents' Night."

"Oh, honey, I knew about that a week ago. The school sent out a letter."

"They did?"

"Sure."

"Why didn't you say anything?"

"I didn't want to go if you didn't want me to."

"But I do want you to go, Grandma."

"It's OK, Valerie. I know you want your mother to go with you."

All of a sudden I knew that I really did want Grandma to go. I wasn't just saying it to make her feel good.

"Grandma," I told her, "I want you to come because you really are my mother. I mean, you're the one who takes care of me."

"No, Valerie. I'm not your mother. You have a mother, and she'll always be your mother. And that's fine. But I am something else that's very special to you, too."

"What's that, Grandma?"

"I'm your family."

I just stood there then until she pointed to the table and we both sat down.

"I wish I hadn't called my mother at all," I told her.

"No, honey. I'm glad you did. Because she's so unlucky."

"Unlucky?"

"Sure. She doesn't have you. She doesn't get to look at the clock every day and know you'll be home soon. She doesn't get to help you pick your clothes or watch you eat the food she cooks."

"But Grandma, you have to watch me do my blood checks and give me my insulin, and make healthy foods and everything."

"Oh, I never said it was easy. But that diabetes is part of you. It's like your black hair or your pretty eyes. And I see you getting more grown up every day, doing your blood checks, learning to take your own shots, and I say to myself, 'What a big lady she's becoming.'"

Grandma smiled at me. "You think I gave you a place to live, Valerie, but you gave me a whole new world."

I sat there pushing my fork around my plate and piling my mashed potatoes onto my peas. I wanted to get up and hug Grandma, but I was thinking how she said I was becoming such a big lady.

After awhile I told her, "You know, Grandma, the school made a big mistake."

"They did?"

"Sure. They said it was Parents' Night. But they were wrong. It's really Family Night."

I waited another minute, and then I didn't care if I was becoming a big lady or not. I ran over and hugged Grandma. And I knew she was glad I did, because of how hard she hugged me back.

Bobby Goes to Bat

by Peter Banks

Even before the umpire shouted "Strike three," anyone could see that Kevin was going to strike out. He had missed a lot of practice, being sick so much. And that meant the Tigers were in the Little League basement. Kevin had been their best hitter.

Bobby was standing behind the backstop with Kevin's dad, Mr. Henderson. He could see how Kevin's dad clenched his fingers each time Kevin swung.

Usually, Mr. Henderson was shouting, "Atta boy!" He was proud of how strong Kevin was, how far he could hit, and how independent he was. Bobby knew Mr. Henderson liked that word "independent."

He was always saying, "We Henderson men, we've always been the independent kind." It meant that he and Kevin were supposed to take care of things on their own.

Last year, Kevin's mom and dad had gotten divorced. Now Mr. Henderson lived two towns away. Still, he came to all of Kevin's games, and most weekends Kevin went to his house. Mr. Henderson was always telling Kevin what a big boy he was to understand the divorce, and to take care of his diabetes so well.

Except lately, Kevin's diabetes had been taking care of him, instead of the other way around. Dr. Gordon said he had never seen a case like it. Kevin did all the right things—checked his blood glucose and took his insulin at the right times, and ate healthy foods. But his blood sugar was still as high as a fly ball.

Before, Kevin had usually made one or two home runs

a game. But ever since his diabetes had gotten out of control and he started spending so much time at the doctor's
office, it seemed as if he could barely tap the ball past the
shortstop. Today, the way Kevin dropped the bat and
walked so slowly to where Bobby and Mr. Henderson
were standing, he looked like an old man.

Kevin was Bobby's best friend. When Bobby's family
had moved to West Haven two years ago, it was Kevin
who made him feel at home. Bobby was terrible at sports,
but every day Kevin practiced with him until he got so
good he actually made the Little League team.

And, of course, Kevin had diabetes, just like Bobby.
Kevin was the first one who made Bobby feel as if it were
no big deal. The first time Bobby stayed for dinner at
Kevin's house, he pulled out his syringes and nobody
made a big deal of it. For the first time in his life, Bobby
didn't have to answer all of the dumb questions people
have always asked—Why did he have to take shots? Did
they hurt? What was diabetes anyway? Kevin just knew.

Now, Mr. Henderson was driving Bobby and Kevin
back to Kevin's mom's home after the game. Mr.
Henderson reached over and put his hand on his son's
shoulder. "Don't worry, Kevin," he said. "Once you get
this diabetes licked, your game will come back."

Kevin didn't answer.

Bobby sat in the back seat, behind Kevin, and watched
his friend slump lower and lower in the seat as they drove,
until he could hardly see the top of Kevin's head. That was
how sad Kevin seemed to feel about not being able to control his diabetes better.

Bobby couldn't stand it anymore. He was going to find
a way to help Kevin. He had to.

The next day, Bobby went to Kevin's house first thing in the morning. Mrs. Henderson opened the door. "Kevin's not up yet, Bobby," she said. "I was just going to get him, but why don't you do it for me? It's time for his shot and his breakfast."

But when Bobby went into Kevin's room, Kevin was already up and in the shower. He sat down at Kevin's desk to wait for him. Kevin's diabetes supplies were in neat piles in a plastic desk organizer. Bobby sighed. Kevin was so careful about everything. It couldn't be anything he was doing wrong that was making his diabetes go out of control.

Kevin's logbook was lying open in the middle of the desk. Bobby figured that Kevin must have been checking his numbers to see what was wrong.

Bobby didn't mean to look at the book, but it was open, and suddenly something on the page caught his eye, something that didn't make sense.

Kevin had written that he'd checked his blood glucose at 5 o'clock yesterday. But Bobby knew that Kevin had been outside with him then, and that he hadn't done a blood check. Kevin must have made a mistake, Bobby decided.

When Kevin came back into the room, he saw Bobby reading the logbook. "Stop snooping on me," Kevin said. He slammed the book shut.

"I'm sorry," Bobby told him. "I didn't mean to look. It was open." He didn't say anything more while Kevin started dressing.

But after a minute, he added, "I think you made a mistake, Kev."

Kevin pulled his shirt down over his head fast. All of a sudden he looked very upset. "Just drop it, Bobby," he almost shouted.

Bobby didn't say anything. He was scared. He had never seen Kevin act like this before. He watched while Kevin did his blood check and took his shot.

When they were downstairs, Mrs. Henderson invited Bobby to sit at the table while Kevin ate breakfast. Neither of them said anything. "What's wrong with you boys?" Mrs. Henderson asked from the kitchen. "I've never heard you two so quiet before."

Bobby kept looking at Kevin, and Kevin kept staring back, frowning. Then Bobby remembered. There was a time he had annoyed Kevin. It happened the night Kevin had slept over. In the morning, Kevin hadn't taken his insulin. When Bobby asked why, Kevin seemed angry and said it was a new thing Dr. Gordon was trying.

Then Bobby had a funny idea. What if the numbers in Kevin's logbook weren't a mistake? What if Kevin had made them up? And what if Dr. Gordon had never told Kevin to skip his shot? What if he had just done it himself? Wouldn't that make him sick?

As soon as Kevin was finished eating, Bobby said, "Let's play catch." Kevin nodded and went to get his glove.

Outside, Bobby said, "Kev, if I ask you something, promise not to get mad?"

Kevin stopped and looked at Bobby. "Sure," he said. "What's the matter?"

"Kev, are you making your-self sick?"

Kevin smiled, a funny half smile. "You're crazy," he said.

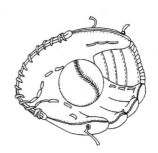

99

"Why would I do that? It's just that Dr. Gordon can't figure things out."

Bobby sighed. "Kevin, I would never tell on you. Promise. But I know you're like your dad says, independent. And I know you don't make mistakes like the one I saw in the book. It's okay if you don't want to tell me, Kev. But maybe I can help you, like you helped me learn to throw."

Kevin looked at Bobby a long time. Then he started walking away, not saying anything. Bobby said, "Wait up," and went after him.

They went three blocks before Kevin finally said, "You know, Bobby, I'm tired. I'm tired of shots. I'm tired of tests, and I'm tired of Dr. Gordon. I've been careful with my diabetes all winter, and now it's summertime and I just want to play."

"I know how it is,'" Bobby said. "Sometimes I feel the same way."

"You're wrong about me," Kevin added. "I'm not like my dad says, independent. I'm as big a baby as there is. I want somebody else to take care of my stupid diabetes for awhile."

"But lots of people could help you, Kev," Bobby said. "Your mom and dad could help."

"Hah," Kevin said. "My dad. You know how he talks. 'The independent Henderson men.' He'd be so disappointed in me."

"Kevin, I asked you for help with my game, and you don't think I'm a baby because I asked, do you?"

Kevin shrugged his shoulders. "No. But it's not the same. You know my dad. I just can't tell him I want help."

For a few weeks after that, Bobby tried to get Kevin to

tell his dad. But every time, Kevin just said he couldn't.

His diabetes wasn't getting any better. In fact, it was getting worse. Kevin had been to Dr. Gordon three times last week.

Bobby felt that if he didn't do something soon, Kevin could really hurt himself. But what could Bobby do? He couldn't tell Kevin's mom and dad. Kevin had to tell someone himself.

Then, as he drove with Kevin and Mr. Henderson to the Saturday afternoon game, Bobby thought of something. Maybe Mr. Henderson could tell Kevin it was all right to ask for help, even if he didn't know he was doing it.

"Mr. Henderson," Bobby said. He was sitting in the back seat again. "Could I ask you something?"

"Sure, Bobby," Mr. Henderson said.

"Mr. Henderson, I'm going to quit the team, but I'm afraid to tell my dad."

Mr. Henderson looked over his shoulder at Bobby. Kevin turned around, too. He had a funny look.

"Why would you quit?" Mr. Henderson asked. "You worked so hard. I knew you when you could hardly throw at all. Now, you have a mean curve ball, and I'm not just saying that."

Bobby tried not to smile. His plan was working.

"I'm tired of playing ball," Bobby said. "It's too hard for me. I'm not a good player like Kevin. I'm tired of practice. I'm tired of catching. I'm tired of trying when I know I'll never be any good."

Kevin looked hard at Bobby. "You'd better stop."

Mr. Henderson didn't seem to hear Kevin. "Lots of people would help you practice, Bobby," he said. "I know Kevin would, and I would. And what about your dad? I bet

101

if you told him how you feel he would help you with your game."

"Hah, my dad," Bobby said. "He thinks I'm tough. He was so proud of me when I made the team. I can't tell him I need help. He'd think I was weak."

Mr. Henderson pulled into the ballfield parking lot. Bobby could see kids from the team warming up.

Mr. Henderson turned sideways in his seat to talk to Bobby. Kevin just looked straight out the window.

"Bobby, when your dad says you're tough, that doesn't mean you can't ask him for help," Kevin's dad said. "Take the Henderson men. We're the independent kind. But we ask for help. Independent guys, tough guys, we get help when we need it. When something's bothering Kevin, he's not afraid to tell me. You shouldn't be afraid to talk to your dad."

That was what Bobby wanted to hear. He said, "Is that right? You wouldn't be afraid to talk to your dad?"

Kevin didn't turn around, but Bobby heard him say in a clear, quiet voice, "That's right."

Then Kevin said, "Dad, when Bobby goes to warm up, could we sit here a minute?" Then, softer, he added "I want to talk to you about something."

Bobby slipped out of the car and went to where the other kids were standing. He looked back to the car. He could see Mr. Henderson lean in close to Kevin.

"What's the matter with Kevin?" someone called. "Is he OK?"

Bobby smiled. "He's OK now. In fact, it looks like the Tigers might be getting out of the basement."

Get Out of My Face!

by Marcia Levine Mazur

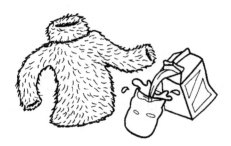

I have a problem—big time. My mother won't get out of my face. I mean, it's, "Jeremy, did you put your jacket on?" and "Jeremy, go to bed," and "Jeremy, did you drink your milk?"

Then there's my lunch. If they made my mom an astronaut, she'd rocket back at noon just to make sure I ate my lunch. In fact, one day I forgot my lunch. So, what does my mom do? She zaps over to the school and gives it to the principal, Ms. Hanrahan. She probably said something like, "My son, Jeremy, absolutely has to have his lunch on time."

So, old Hanrahan goes bonkers and tells a hall guard to bring it to me, and the hall guard turns out to be Anita Cooper—I mean, THE ANITA COOPER—you know, the girl with the blond hair who does you a favor if she says, "Hello."

Anyway, Anita comes flying into old Mr. Prescott's room and tells him—real loud—that my mother says I absolutely have to have my lunch on time. Then the class gets to watch Anita cruise over and plop the lunch bag onto my desk like it was a Scud missile.

Then that night when I told Mom that I wish she hadn't brought my lunch to school, she only said, "Well, you know you do have to eat on time, Jeremy."

Actually, she's right. See, I have this thing called diabetes. It means my body doesn't use food the way it should, so I have to take shots every day—called insulin—and check my blood with a little machine about the size of a pocket calculator. And my Mom's right about eating my meals on time.

Still, ever since we found out I have diabetes, my mother won't get out of my face. I mean, it's been over a year now and she practically guards the door if I reach for the doorknob without a hat on. Sometimes Dad tells her, "Give the boy a chance."

Anyhow, that's why the mess started last week, all because my mom is always in my face. It happened like this. Ms. Hanrahan announced the all-city school picnic, including a baseball game—our Wolverines against the John Adams School Dodgers—and a barbecue lunch. It sounded really cool. I was even chosen to pitch the first three innings for the Wolverines, and then, wham! They asked parents to come, and who signs up? You got it. My mother.

I could just imagine it. I'd be starting my windup, and my mother would be on the foul line waving my sweater at me. Or I'd be eating barbecue, and she'd be running over with my milk.

I mean, do you think Dracula's mother followed him around, telling him, "Drac, drink your blood?" So, all of a sudden I didn't want to go to the picnic at all. I thought about explaining how I felt to Dad, or even to Mom, but I didn't know how to say it. So, I came up with my Secret Master Plan: Get sick.

The week before the picnic, I started sneezing. I knew I'd have to stay in bed all day Sunday if they thought I was sick, but that was better than going to the picnic with Mom.

Problem was, it wasn't working. I was sneezing away big time, but she wasn't buying it. She didn't suspect, or anything, but the picnic was Sunday, and by Friday morning all she said was, "I hope you're not getting sick, Jeremy."

She did call the doctor Friday afternoon when I came home from school. And you know what the doctor told her? "Keep an eye on him." That's like telling Babe Ruth to hit a home run. It just comes naturally.

Anyhow, by Saturday noon my mother and I were still on for the picnic and I was getting nervous. I mean, she's a nice mother and all, but I knew that picnic was going to be awful—big time.

So, after lunch, I stayed at the table waiting for something to happen. And it did. Dad asked me if I wanted to pitch a few. When I whispered, "I don't think so," Mom said I was sick.

"Jeremy, I hate to tell you this, but I don't think you're going to that picnic tomorrow."

I pretended to be surprised. "But, Mom, I'm OK."

"Well, better safe than sorry." That's one of her favorites, "Better safe than sorry." She felt my forehead. "You go to bed and I'll bring you some diet soda."

"You going to be OK, boy?" Dad asked me.

"Sure," I said, and gave them a sick cough. I shut my

bedroom door, got into my pajamas, and hopped into bed.

But things started to go bad when Mom came in with the diet soda. She looked so sad and sat on the bed and stroked my forehead. She even kissed me on the cheek. "I'm sorry you're sick. Jeremy."

Then she switched off the light and tiptoed out.

That's when the real pain started. All of a sudden I was really hurting. . .only not my chest or my throat, but inside. I felt terrible, pretending like that, fooling them. After all, I know Mom gets in my face so much 'cause she loves me.

I buried my face in the pillow. It felt funny to be in bed in the middle of the day, especially when I felt fine. Except that I didn't feel fine. I felt awful.

I couldn't understand it. The Master Plan had worked. I had what I wanted. Only now I didn't want it—not this way. But, I still didn't want my mom at the school picnic.

I didn't know what to do. I just closed my eyes and I fell asleep. When I woke up, it was dinner time.

I took my insulin and then we ate, but no one talked, except Mom, of course. She kept pushing the lima beans at me, saying, "Eat. They're good for you."

Afterwards, I curled up in the big chair in the family room, and Mom came over and wrapped a blanket around me. She turned on the TV, sat down on the sofa, and curled her feet under her. Dad was in the armchair.

Then I had an idea. I threw back the blanket, ran into the kitchen, poured a glass of milk, and brought it to her. She looked at me funny. "This is nice of you, Jeremy, but I've just had supper."

"Well, you look thirsty," I told her. And then I went to the hall closet and got her red sweater. "Better put it on,

Mom."

"That's very sweet of you, Jeremy." She looked confused, but slipped on the sweater. I sat down and pulled
the blanket around me.

But a minute later I bopped up again, dragged Mom
and Dad's quilt in from their bedroom and covered Mom
with it the way she had covered me.

"I'm not chilly, Jeremy."

"Well, you look chilly," I said.

"Why should I be chilly? It's perfectly warm in here."

"Well, you covered me with a blanket. Why should I
be chilly?"

"Richard," she turned to my dad, "Do you think he's
having an insulin reaction?"

"I think he's just telling us that he knows when he's
thirsty or cold," Dad said softly.

"But we have to take special care of him. He has diabetes."

"But that doesn't mean I don't know when I'm cold,
Mom!"

She looked at me like she had met me on Mars—you
know, that time when they made her an astronaut. "Mom,
it's OK if you help me with my insulin shots and blood
checks sometimes. But I wish you wouldn't worry about
everything else all the time."

Then she started to cry—big time. Dad put his arms
around her, and I wanted my chair seat to break so I could
just fall through. I started thinking about a TV series they
could make out of me, "The Boy Who Made His Mother
Cry."

After awhile Mom said, "Jeremy, is all this so I'll let
you go to the picnic tomorrow?"

"Heck no. I don't even want to go to the picnic," I told her.

"But why not?"

Here it was. If I didn't tell her how I felt now, then some day I'd be the only kid in college whose mother still brought him his lunch.

"Well," I took a deep breath. "I really do want to go to the picnic. But not if you're going to tell me to wear my jacket or drink my milk in front of the other kids. So I said I was sick."

Dad looked at me in a kind of surprised way. "Guess the boy has a mind of his own." I wanted to tell him to stop calling me "the boy," but I figured that could wait til next time. Good thinking, too, 'cause he got Mom to stop crying.

Finally, she stood up, all stiff-looking and said, "We're very upset that you weren't truthful, Jeremy, but since I promised I'd go the picnic, you can go, too. And don't worry, I'll pretend I don't even know you."

I felt awful, but Dad squeezed my shoulder and said why didn't I go take my snack and get a good night's sleep? "Tomorrow's going to be a big day."

Boy, he was right about that. In fact, it turned out to be a much bigger day than I expected. It started when Mom and I got on the school bus.

First off, she made such a fuss about not sitting next to me that I kept smacking my baseball into my glove so I didn't have to talk to anyone until we got there. I really felt bad.

Then when we got to the park, she stood far away from me when Ms. Hanrahan gave instructions. "A bell will ring promptly at 4:00. When you hear the bell, you have fifteen minutes to get back to the bus."

Then Mom turned and went off with the other mothers. I stopped thinking about all the trouble with my mother and everything went great. The Wolverines won the game and the other team's coach said I was the best pitcher he'd ever seen in my age group.

I looked for Mom at lunchtime, but she stayed far away and ate with the other mothers. But at 4:00 the real problem started. The bell rang, like they said it would, and—get this—I couldn't find my mother! I was a little scared. I mean, was she so mad she just went off by herself? Then they found out that four mothers were missing!

Ms. Hanrahan sent out a search party and the rest of us waited at the buses. To tell you the truth, I walked around to the other side of the bus because I didn't want the guys to see how bad I felt.

All of a sudden the search party came charging back and behind them were the four mothers. Turns out the mothers were playing cards at a table on the other side of the park and didn't hear the bell. Would you believe?

All that was five months ago now, but I still kid Mom about it, especially when she starts getting in my face with the sweaters and milk and stuff. But that doesn't happen so much anymore.

She and Dad see that I really can take care of myself. And they know how I feel, so I'm glad I told them, even if it was kind of a nutty way to do it.

Besides, now Mom and I keep talking about next year's picnic, as if all the bad stuff hadn't even happened. We talk about how we're both going to have fun there— big time.

PLEASE LISTEN, DAD...

By Marcia Levine Mazur

He just won't watch," Vicky said. It was noon on Saturday, and she and her friend, Bea, were hurrying home from the library. "I mean, he walks away every time."

"Your father?"

"Yes! My own father." Vicky shook her head.

"He thinks I don't notice. But he's never there when I take my insulin injection. He won't even watch me do a blood glucose check. I mean, Mom watches me, but not him." Vicky took a deep breath and walked faster.

"What's his problem?" Bea asked, trying to keep up.

"My diabetes."

"But that's your problem."

"I know!"

"That's weird."

"No it isn't." Vicky didn't like anyone, even her best friend, calling her father weird.

The girls came to their grey brick apartment building and bounced up the steps. Bea opened the door to number 16, and waved. Vicky headed for her own home, apartment 38.

"Hi, honey, what do you have there?" Since it was Saturday, Dad was home, sitting at the kitchen table reading the paper as Vicky walked in.

"Library books. Bea and I are going to read *Little Women* 'cause we liked the movie so much."

"Good for you."

Mom was just closing the oven door and Vicky could

110

sniff the lasagna inside. "Lunch coming up," Mom announced.

Vicky knew what that meant. She set the books down, headed for her diabetes drawer, and took out her kit. Dad stood, gave a funny kind of cough, and announced, "I think I left the sports page in the living room."

Vicky watched him walk out. "You know, it really hurts that he won't watch me do my glucose check or take an injection."

"I know," Mom said. "It's taking a long time for him to get used to your diabetes."

"Well, I had to get used to it pretty fast," Vicky snapped. Then she was sorry she'd said that. So she added, "Isn't there anything we can do to help him?"

"I'm afraid not, honey. I guess he just needs more time."

Dad came back just as Vicky was putting her supplies away, and the three of them sat down. Mom spooned the steaming lasagna onto their plates, and set a pile of bright green string beans next to it. They all had milk.

No one talked. You could hear the chewing, and Vicky wanted to laugh out loud.

But it wasn't funny. So much of their time together had been like this—quiet. No one talking. It had started when they found out she had diabetes, and that was six months ago!

Vicky was scraping the last forkful of lasagna from her plate when Bea knocked. Vicky did laugh out loud this time. Bea looked like she'd just landed on earth from outer space. She had her knee pads and helmet on, and her skateboard under her arm.

"Got your board?" she asked.

"Sure," Vicky set her dish in the sink, went to her room, and came back wearing her own knee pads and helmet. She headed for the door, carrying her skateboard under her left arm.

"Rub sun block on," Dad called, you can't be too careful. . . ."

Vicky rolled her eyes at Bea. She knew Dad wanted to say, "You can't be too careful when you have diabetes." She also knew that he didn't finish his sentence because he never said that word, 'diabetes.'

About a week ago, she had figured out why he never said it. It was because it must seem to him that if he never said, 'diabetes,' then she didn't really have it.

Vicky and Bea ran down the steps and set their skateboards onto a cement path in the back of the building. Then they rolled them back and forth a few times to make sure the wheels worked well.

Old Mrs. Rose, who waddled when she walked, was sitting on a bench. Vicky and Bea smiled at her.

Mrs. Rose smiled back. "My, you have pretty eyes," she said to Vicky, and Vicky felt her cheeks burn from embarrassment. "What do you call that color?"

"They're hazel. It's a kind of greenish-brown," Vicky called, skating away.

She and Bea did a couple of slow laps around the path. Then they tried some fancy stuff. Suddenly Vicky's skate rolled right out from under her and she fell hard.

Bea was there in a minute. "You OK?" she asked.

"Sure. It's just my ankle."

"I'll go get your momma," Mrs. Rose called, waddling off. Her walk was so funny that Bea and Vicky couldn't help laughing. But Vicky stopped quickly. "Ooooo, it hurts."

"What happened?" Dad was there faster than she thought Mrs. Rose could waddle up the stairs. Mom rushed up a minute later.

"What's wrong?" Dad asked again. Are you hurt?"

"I'm fine. Fine." Vicky answered. "Just twisted my ankle."

"I'll bring the car around and we'll take you to the emergency room," Dad told her.

"It's not that bad," Vicky answered, although she was in pain.

"You can't be too careful," he began, "you know. . . ."

"I know. I know. I have diabetes." Vicky finished his sentence for him. But Dad was already rushing off for the car.

"He's just so worried about you," Mom told her, bending down to look at Vicky's ankle. "You'll understand when you have kids of your own."

Vicky didn't answer. That was another expression she could live without.

Dad drove the car right up over the grass and onto the cement, then lifted Vicky onto the back seat. Mom scrunched in next to her, and Bea waved as the three of them sped off.

Both Dad and Vicky were right. Dr. Royce said there weren't any broken bones, but that her ankle did need to be bandaged.

Home again. Vicky had dinner, then sat reading *Little Women* until bedtime, her leg resting on a chair. The book, she decided, was definitely neater than the movie.

After her blood glucose check and a snack, Vicky wrapped herself in her old bathrobe—her pajamas didn't go over the bandaged ankle—and tried to sleep.

But her leg throbbed, and about midnight she sat up. Someone was in the kitchen. As quietly as she could, she hobbled over to the kitchen door.

The room was dark. But the moonlight coming through the window showed someone sitting at the table.

Dad! It was Dad, sitting alone in the dark. And the noise was coming from him. Dad was crying!

Vicky slid into the chair next to him. She wanted say, "Please, Dad, stop crying. It scares me."

But she only whispered, "Don't worry. My ankle is fine."

Dad looked at her. "I'm sorry, Vicky. I mean, I'm sorry you have diabetes. I'm so sorry."

"It's not your fault. You didn't give it to me."

"Yes, I did. I mean, no I didn't, not exactly. You know, I'd rather have it a million times instead of you."

"I know," Vicky whispered.

But he didn't seem to be listening. "My grandmother Bessie—my mother's mother—lived with us, and she had diabetes for years. I used to watch her boil those old syringes and use them over and over. And she had to put urine in a little pan on the stove, and dip a special paper in it to see if her diabetes was OK."

"Urine?"

"Yes. Urine. They didn't have those blood glucose gadgets you have today."

"Ugh," Vicky said. "I'm glad I'm living today."

"And then we found out that my father's sister—Aunt Ida—had it, too. And there's no one at all in Mom's family who has diabetes. So you must have gotten it from me."

Vicky was quiet a minute, then she said softly, "Dad?"

"What?" He was looking down at the table.

"I really think that's crazy."

He turned and mussed her hair. "You're too young, Vicky. You don't understand."

She never got anywhere when grownups talked like that, so she said the first thing that came into her mind. "You know, Mrs. Rose told me I had pretty hazel eyes today."

"Well, you do."

"Hey, you know what, Dad? You have hazel eyes, too."

She saw a tiny smile cross his face, and it gave her an idea.

"Dad, you remember when you told me Uncle Arnie could play the piano like a pro? He's your brother, isn't he?"

"Sure is. And he could have been a pro if he wanted," Dad answered.

"Well, the new music teacher, Mrs. Brandon, said I have good musical sense."

"Sure you do. You'll be in the high school orchestra next year."

"Well," Vicky went on excitedly, "Maybe I wouldn't have such good musical sense if it weren't for your family. And maybe I wouldn't have hazel eyes if it weren't for you, and maybe . . . ."

This time Dad leaned way back and shook his head.

"Well, honey, much as I'd like to take credit for all that, I didn't really hand you your hazel eyes or your musical talent. They just happened."

"So did my diabetes."

He sat straight up then. Vicky swallowed, waited a minute, then went on. "Dad, you rushed to take me to the hospital when I hurt my ankle, but you won't even watch

115

me do a blood glucose check. What's so different about diabetes?"

"Honey, I didn't mean. . . ."

Vicky didn't know if she was angry or sad. She decided she was angry.

"I know. I know. It's cause you're sorry I have it. And it's 'cause you think it's your fault 'cause your Grandmother Bessie and your Aunt Ida had diabetes. But how do you think I feel when you walk away, or when you won't talk about it?"

He started to say something, but she hurried on. "I feel like something's really wrong with me. And I know there isn't, because I have all kinds of fun. I go skateboarding, and I go to camp, and I'll be in the school orchestra and . . . and I have hazel eyes," she finished."

Dad stood up, and Vicky was sure he was going to march out of the room again.

But he didn't. Instead, he reached out and put his hands on her shoulders. "You know, you're a pretty terrific kid. And you're pretty smart, too. And I understand what you're saying. It's funny, but my Grandmother Bessie used to say something like that, too. In fact, she heard it from her mother. She said, "In this life, you have to take the bad with the good.

"And," he added, "in your case, the good is very, very, good."

"Same with you, Dad," Vicky answered, looking up at him, forgetting her anger. "Same with you."

Grandmother, Granddaughter

by Marcia Levine Mazur

It was April. Pink and yellow flowers poked through the wet ground, snow melted into puddles, and school closed for spring vacation. But it was a strange time for 12-year old P.D.

Her mother's mother—P.D. always called her Gran— had died a month earlier.

P.D. (actually Pauline Dena) was named for her Gran, but she'd been glad when friends started calling her P.D. "Pauline Dena is so old fashioned," she told everyone. "And P.D. is so neat."

Although she'd known for months that Gran was sick, she was still surprised when Mom and Dad came into her room that rainy morning, hugged her, and said softly, "Honey, Gran passed away last night."

She knew what that meant. Gran had died.

Mom cried a lot at first—especially at the funeral. Gran was buried in their local cemetary, but now there was so much to do at Gran's house And, since school was out, Mom wanted P.D. to fly to Cleveland with her and help go through Gran's things. "Maybe you'll find something of Gran's you'd like to keep," she said.

"What would I want of Gran's?" P.D. thought, but she didn't say it out loud.

When her friend Colleen came over later to practice jump shots, P.D. told her, "Mom and I are going to Cleveland tomorrow to see about Gran's stuff."

"But what about practice?" Colleen wailed. "We'll never make the team if we don't practice."

Colleen and P.D. were starting junior high in the fall, and both wanted to make the freshman basketball team.

"Well, it's not my fault. I don't want to go to Cleveland," P.D. answered, dribbling the ball around the yard. "1 mean, it's not like I really knew Gran. She lived so far away and we only visited her a couple of times a year. I don't even know what she did for fun." She stooped, aimed, and sank the ball.

P.D. didn't tell Colleen the other reason she didn't want to go. It was because of the loneliness she knew she'd find in Gran's house. It would be difficult to walk up those porch steps and into the front door and not have Gran there to hug her, show her how to knead the bread, or ask her to serve the big white platter of steaming chicken.

P.D. remembered last year when everyone sat waiting around the huge dining room table. Then she had come in from the kitchen carrying the food. They had all started to clap. Of course, she knew they were clapping because Gran's food was so good, but she also knew that she was a part of it all.

P.D. wished now that she had talked to Gran about real things when they were together, not just about how to knead bread or spoon food onto a platter. She would have gotten to know Gran that way. But it was too late now, and P.D. didn't want to go back into that big empty house.

"I have an idea how to get out of the trip," she told Colleen while they bounced the ball back and forth.

"What?"

"You'll see.

That night at dinner P.D. announced that the flight to Cleveland might send her diabetes out of control. (P.D. had been diagnosed with diabetes three years earlier, and she knew Mom and Dad still worried about her.)

"Why should that happen?" Dad asked, looking up from his plate. "Flying doesn't hurt diabetes."

P.D. wanted to say, "How do you know? You and Mom don't have diabetes." But she just forked in another mouthful of corn.

Mom's eyes teared up, and P.D. knew she was thinking about Gran again. But she surprised P.D. by saying, "You know, Gran was so proud to have a granddaughter."

"She was?" P.D. asked, forgetting to chew the corn. She'd never thought much about being a granddaughter.

"It's too bad you didn't get to know her well," Mom answered. "She was quite a woman."

"I guess we didn't talk much because she didn't speak English well," P.D. said, chewing again.

"Gran always wished she could speak English better. But it's hard to change languages when you're born in another country," Mom told her.

P.D. nodded. "I can't even imagine moving and having to learn a new language," she said. But she didn't add the main reason she hadn't talked to Gran about anything much. It was because she didn't know what to say to old people.

Looking at Mom, P.D. realized how much her mother wanted her to go to Cleveland with her. "I'll get packed," P.D. said, leaving the table.

"We can practice our jump shots all summer," she kept

explaining to Colleen on the phone later.

The flight to Cleveland was fun, but an hour after they landed, Mom was unlocking the door to Gran's house.

It was dark and a little scary inside. P.D. flipped on the lights, and they walked into the flowered kitchen. Gran's old black stove stood on its four legs, and P.D. thought it looked lonely. "I bet it misses Gran," she said.

"So many wonderful meals my mother made on this old thing," Mom almost whispered, smoothing her hand across it. "Her roast chicken was so tender the meat fell off the bones. Remember? And the fish! No one could get enough of her fish. And those potatoes. They sat in the oven all night and got so brown and crusty. I guess we'll never eat potatoes like that again."

P.D. remembered the potatoes, and the chicken, and the fish. But mostly she remembered Gran's fresh loaves of braided bread.

"I have to make a phone call," Mom said. "Why don't you start in the bedroom and I'll be right there?"

The bedroom door creaked as P.D. opened it and flicked on the light. It didn't feel right to be there. Whenever they had visited, Mom or Dad would tell her to stay out of Gran's room. Now she and Mom were going to look all through it.

She walked over to the dresser. What was in those drawers she'd never been allowed to open?

P.D. tugged at the small top drawer and it slid out. The whole drawer smelled like flowers. There were three shiny rings and a pin on top of a pile of white handkerchiefs. P.D. tried one ring on. It fit perfectly. "I guess Gran and I are the same size," she thought, putting the ring back. Maybe she'd ask Mom for the ring as her souvenir. But she certainly didn't want the handkerchiefs.

"Why would anybody keep them?" she wondered. "Tissues are so easy. You just throw them away."

She shut the small drawer and looked into the larger one in the middle.

There were two neat piles of flannel nightgowns there, so old they were almost worn through. She pictured her own shorty Disney P.J.s and almost slammed the drawer shut.

The huge bottom drawer opened easily, and it held the prize. Photograph albums.

P.D. lugged the biggest onto Gran's high soft bed, climbed onto the feather-filled quilt, and opened the book.

There was a picture of an old fashioned family, a mother sitting in a chair, three children in long, white dresses leaning on her, and a stiff-looking man standing next to the chair.

The oldest child looked familiar. Gran? Was that Gran? Gran with her Mom and Dad?

P.D. turned the page carefully, then whistled. Gran again, only this time in a wedding dress! P.D. knew Gran was married, of course, but Grandpa had died years ago. Now here was the grandmother she remembered, only she was young and pretty.

The next picture was the shocker. P.D. could tell it was taken later than the others, but Gran was still young. This time she was on a sandy beach, standing up, and smiling. And Gran was wearing a black bathing suit, even if it did come almost to her knees!

"Imagine Gran swimming!" P.D. thought. "Maybe that's what she did for fun when she was young. Swim. Just like me."

121

Mom came in then, ready to work, but P.D. held out the picture. "Look, here's Gran in a bathing suit."

Mom looked at the photo briefly. "She loved to swim," she said. Then she turned to the window and started to laugh.

"What's so funny?" P.D. asked.

"Mrs. Green."

"Who's Mrs. Green?"

"She used to live next door and she would get these really enormous hiccups. They were so loud you could actually hear them in here through all the walls."

"What happened?"

"Well, the first time we brought you for a visit—you were a tiny baby—we put you to sleep in here and then Mrs. Green started hiccuping. Gran was so angry."

P.D. curled up on the bed, "Why was she angry?"

"She thought the hiccups would wake you, so she banged on the window, but Mrs. Green didn't hear."

"She was afraid I'd wake up?" P.D. repeated, pleased.

"Sure. So she filled a glass of water and stormed over to Mrs. Green's. She wanted Mrs. Green to drink the water and stop hiccuping. Only when Mrs. Green opened the door, she let out a big hiccup. Instead of getting her to stop, Gran began hiccuping, too! After that, the two of them couldn't stop laughing—or hiccupping."

Mom started laughing again. P.D. liked the story. She liked to think of Gran marching over to Mrs. Green's, getting the hiccups, and laughing about it. She would have laughed too, she was sure. But sitting here laughing now seemed wrong.

"Mom," she asked softly, "how can you laugh in Gran's room now?"

Mom sat down next to her daughter and put her arm

around her. "Just because people die doesn't mean you can't remember the good times you had with them. In fact, that helps keep them alive inside your heart."

"It does?" P.D. asked. She leaned on Mom's shoulder and after a minute she added, "I wish I knew Gran better. She seems pretty neat."

Suddenly Mom stood up again. "I guess I didn't know her as well as I thought either. I found a bottle of diabetes pills in the medicine chest. They were dated three months ago! She must have been diagnosed in January, and she never even told me. I'm so annoyed. Why didn't she tell me?"

All at once P.D. realized something amazing. She understood better than Mom or Dad or anyone why Gran never told them she had diabetes. P.D. had not wanted to tell anyone either.

"Gran didn't tell you because she didn't want you to think there was anything wrong with her," P.D. said.

"Really? How do you know?" Mom asked, still annoyed.

"Because Gran and I both have diabetes."

Mom looked at her for a second, then nodded, "Yes, I guess you do."

"Mom," P.D. added, "I think I know what I'd like to take for a souvenir of Gran."

"One of those rings?"

"Well, one of them was pretty nice. And it fit. But what I really want is to take her name again."

"Pauline Dena? But you said it was old fashioned."

"Well, maybe not the whole name. Maybe just Paulie, like people sometimes called Gran."

"That's nice," Mom said. "But why would you want to

do that?"

"Because it would make Gran happy."

"How do you know?"

"Because I know Gran. We're a lot alike. After all, I am her granddaughter."

Brothers, Sisters

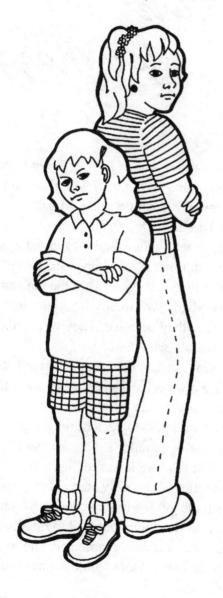

Making Time for Maggie

by Peter Banks

Jennifer couldn't wait for Alison and her Mom to come. She was going shopping at the mall with them to pick out a birthday present for her little sister, Maggie. Maggie would be eight on Tuesday.

She stood at the front window and looked out again, for about the twentieth time. Please hurry, she thought. I've got to get out of here. Maggie was in the kitchen with Mom and Dad. Everybody was totally freaking out. Jennifer hated the way they sounded. They were talking about her like she wasn't even there.

Maggie was crying, saying how they only paid attention to Jennifer. "We always have to eat when she eats! We can only have stuff that she can have!"

It almost made Jennifer's stomach hurt to hear Maggie talk. It was all because of Jennifer's diabetes that everybody was yelling. She felt like it was all her fault.

Maggie was shouting. "You only care about Jennifer. You don't even help me get ready for school anymore."

Jennifer could hear her Mom and Dad saying that wasn't true. But she knew it was. Jennifer remembered how before she got diabetes, Mom would always brush

Maggie's hair before school. Maggie had fine blond hair, just like Madonna, and everybody said how neat it was.

But after Jennifer got diabetes, Mom forgot about Maggie's hair. She had to watch Jennifer do her blood check. She was always nervous, asking things like "Did you get a big enough drop of blood, Jennifer," or "Don't forget to write down the number, Jennifer."

Mom was so nervous it made Jennifer nervous, too. Dad wasn't any better. He used to take Maggie to her soccer games. He played soccer in college and he really liked to yell a lot when Maggie made a goal. Or at least he used to. Now when Jennifer and Dad went to watch Maggie's soccer games, he spent most of his time asking Jennifer if she felt alright, was she sure she felt alright?

Half the time when Maggie scored and turned around to wave to him, he wasn't even looking at the field. He was looking at Jennifer.

It was no wonder Maggie was so mad all the time. It was like she was invisible all of a sudden, and Mom and Dad couldn't see her anymore.

Today, what had gotten Maggie so mad was Mom making plans for her birthday dinner at home. "I thought we could have dinner around 6, because that's when Jennifer has to eat," Mom said. "And we could make a special cake so Jennifer can have some, too."

When Mom said that, Maggie almost exploded. "It's my party! I don't care about Jennifer and her stupid diabetes!"

It was getting like this all the time, Jennifer thought. Maggie was always mad at her, because Mom and Dad seemed to pay so much attention to her these days. But what could Jennifer do about it? She couldn't make her diabetes just go away. And she couldn't make Mom and Dad pay attention to Maggie.

Alison's Mom's car pulled up outside and Jennifer called, "Bye. Alison's here." Maggie was still crying and her Mom and Dad were both talking.

It was good to get into the car with Alison and her Mom. Alison was Jennifer's best friend and she could always make her laugh.

"How's it going, Jennifer babes," Alison said as she slid over to make room on the front seat for Jennifer. She was always saying things like that. "You think we'll see Scott Adelman at the mall?"

"Alison, you are not going to go prowling the mall for boys," Mrs. Walker said.

"Prowling?" Alison said. She leaned her head back on the seat and laughed. "Prooowling, Mom? Is that what they did when you were our age, back in olden times?"

"You know what I mean, Alison Marie," Mrs. Walker said. "We're there to shop."

Alison looked at Jennifer. "Shop till you drop," they said together and laughed out loud.

Alison's favorite thing to do was to go clothes shopping. Alison had nine pairs of shoes, not counting running shoes (she had three pairs of those).

Mrs. Walker kept complaining about how many clothes Alison had. The thing was, though, Mrs. Walker liked to shop just as much as Alison did. They were a lot alike, really, the same laugh, the same smile, the way they both made you feel happy.

But the best thing about Alison and Mrs. Walker was that they didn't make a big deal about Jennifer's diabetes. She could give herself a shot at the Walker's house and nobody asked questions after the first time she showed them.

At home, Mom and Dad looked at Jennifer as if all they saw was her diabetes. At the Walker's house, everybody looked at Jennifer and saw Jennifer, who happened to have diabetes just like she happened to have blue eyes and brown hair. Maybe if things were like that at home, Maggie wouldn't be such a space case all the time.

At the mall, Alison went wild, as usual. She could look through more clothes faster than anybody. She got mad in the stores where they only let you try on three things at a time, because it slowed her down too much.

Mrs. Walker tried to help Jennifer find a present for Maggie. Nothing seemed right: not sweaters, not toys, not books. Whatever Jennifer gave her, Maggie would probably throw back in her face and say "You can keep your stupid present, I don't want it," as if it were Jennifer's fault for having diabetes.

By the time they got halfway through the mall, Jennifer felt sad again. Not even being with Alison made her feel better—not even when Alison practically fell on the floor when she really did see Scott Adelman in Burger Heaven.

Finally, while Alison was trying on a pink miniskirt, Mrs. Walker asked her if something was wrong.

Jennifer bit her lip. "I don't know. I mean, it's Maggie. I think she really hates me. She even put a line of string down the middle of our room and told me never to come on her side. She won't sit next to me at dinner."

"Sisters can be pretty mean like that sometimes," Mrs. Walker said. "It doesn't mean anything."

"But it's because of my diabetes," Jennifer blurted out.

"Maggie's mad because Mom and Dad are always paying attention to me. I feel like it's my fault sometimes."

"It's nobody's fault, Jennifer. Your Mom and Dad love you and they want to make sure you're safe. That's why they spend so much time with you."

Mrs. Walker leaned closer. "Listen, you've already given Maggie a lot by acting so grown up about your diabetes. I don't know if I could do all the things you do, and Alison says I'm practically an old lady. It's just going to take some time and then they'll feel like they can relax. Then they'll have more time for Maggie and she'll be okay."

Mrs. Walker was right, of course. It was going to take time. Jennifer wished her life was like a tape that you could run on fast forward. Then you could skip over the part where Maggie was so mad and get to the part where everybody was happy again.

Alison came out of the dressing room, wearing the pink miniskirt. "Don't tell me you're talking about Mag the Drag again."

Mrs. Walker looked up and her eyes got really wide. "Alison Marie, you are not going to school in that."

Alison rolled her eyes at Jennifer. "But it's so totally cute."

Later, Mrs. Walker bought them lunch. They both got big salads with tiny pink shrimp. Alison said she read somewhere that shrimp made your hair get shinier. Alison kept talking through lunch and Jennifer nodded.

But all the time she kept thinking about what Mrs. Walker had said. She knew it wasn't her fault that Maggie was mad. Still, there had to be a way to make time for Maggie.

It wasn't until two days later, Maggie's birthday, that Jennifer decided what she was going to get Maggie.

She went to the store with Alison after school to get it. Alison couldn't understand the present. "But wouldn't Mag like clothes better?" she asked. "Everybody likes clothes, even Mag the Drag."

But Mrs. Walker smiled. She understood. "I think it's perfect, Jennifer."

But Jennifer wasn't so sure it was perfect when Maggie had finished opening all of Mom and Dad's presents.

"Maggie," Jennifer said. "This is for you, but I have to give it to Mom and Dad."

She handed the present to Dad.

"For us?" Dad said. "You want us to open it?"

Jennifer nodded.

Dad pulled off the wrapping paper and folded it. He was always so slow and careful, it made everybody crazy. He liked them to reuse the paper, so he didn't tear it.

He took out the little black book. "A 'Week at a Glance' book," he said to Mom. "For planning our week."

He handed it to Mom. She turned it over in her hand. "Jennifer, it's so nice, but why . . . "

Jennifer took a deep breath. "Open to the first page."

Together Mom and Dad turned to the place where Jennifer had written in things to do.

"I wanted to give Maggie time with you when you didn't have to worry about me," she said. "I hope it's not too dumb or anything.

"I put down that date for you, Mom, at 7 o'clock in the morning. Brush Maggie's hair. Dad can help me do my blood glucose check while you're doing that."

"And Dad, for you I wrote in 2 o'clock Saturday. Maggie's game. I think Mom and I could do something else, because you're the one that likes soccer so much."

They were all staring at her, Mom, Dad, and Maggie, too. She wanted to run and hide. It was a dumb present.

Maggie was the first one to say anything. "I'm sorry for being a brat, Jen. You can come on my side of the room, anytime, I promise. I'll get rid of the string."

Mom and Dad looked funny. Mom looked like she might cry. "We're sorry, too, Jen," Dad said.

Mom said softly, "I guess sometimes kids are smarter than their parents. We worried about your diabetes so much we forgot about Maggie sometimes. Thank you for helping us to remember."

Then Mom pulled her close and gave her a hug.

"Don't step on the wrapping paper!" Dad said. They all laughed.

Maggie looked at her watch. "It's 6 o'clock," Maggie said. "Time for Jennifer to eat. We should have dinner now. And Jennifer can sit by me."

Don't Mess with the Bryant Brothers

by Marcia Levine Mazur

Want to know the best thing about me? That's easy. It's my big brother, Greg! He's taller and better looking. He's on the basketball team, and he even lifts weights.

Want to know the worst thing about me? That's easy, too. My height. I'm so short, teachers put me in the front row so I can see the blackboard, even though I'm in the seventh grade now. And last year when they took our class picture and the photographer said, "Who's that sitting down in the back?" everybody yelled out, "That's Danny, and he's not sitting!"

Another thing, sometimes bigger guys kind of pick on me, but only the ones who don't know about my brother, Greg. Like that time that new kid Billy Frazer grabbed my lunch bag in the schoolyard and took a bite of my apple.

Greg was way over by the basketball court, but he saw it. A minute later he was standing next to me with one hand on my shoulder, kind of like we were one person.

He held the other hand straight out toward Billy and when Billy saw how quiet everyone was, he just set that apple in Greg's hand. Then he spit out the bite right into his own hand. It must have felt pretty yucky.

Greg stared at him hard. "Don't mess with the Bryant brothers," he said. "You got that? I mean, you really got that?" Billy nodded and walked away. He was still carrying his apple bite. I guess he forgot he had it. Then Greg and I did our "high five" routine.

Like I said, the best thing about me is my big brother.

Or, it used to be, because something happened to Greg. He got sick, so sick they put him in the hospital.

It was hard to believe. I mean, if you wanted to draw a picture of what it looks like not to be sick, you'd draw my big brother, Greg.

Then one afternoon he fell off his bike . . . didn't hit the curb or anything, just fell off. I started to help him, but he shoved me away. I think he was mad at himself for falling—and maybe at me for seeing him fall.

At dinnertime Mom asked him what was wrong, because he didn't seem to be his old self lately. Dad asked him if he was off his feed.

I thought that was funny, because Greg was on his feed pretty good. In fact, he was eating everything in sight. Drinking, too. He stood at the sink and gulped five glasses of water—you could hear them go down, glug, glug. Then he brought another glass to the table.

He had to go to the bathroom a lot, too. I know. We share a bedroom, and I heard his bare feet slapping down the hall three times that night.

Even Mom and Dad must have heard him going to the bathroom, because the next day they made an emergency appointment and took him to the clinic. They asked old Mrs. Carvelli from next door to kind of keep me company, and she tried to talk to me, but, let's face it, Mrs. Carvelli and I haven't got a lot to talk about.

So we both sat and watched TV—but the house felt so empty, even the TV couldn't drown out the quiet. I couldn't wait for Greg to come home.

Only he didn't. I mean, not that night. Dad called about 6 o'clock and said they were at the hospital, and for Mrs. Carvelli to fix some sandwiches. When Mom and Dad came in later, they said Greg would be in the hospital a few nights. He had something called diabetes.

I was really scared then. I looked at Greg's empty bed, and almost cried. Maybe I did cry a little. I missed him. I even missed the sound of his bare feet slapping down to the bathroom.

You can imagine how surprised everyone at school was. They all hung around me like I was really popular, especially Adele—who only talks to me to ask about Greg. She asked me over and over, "What does Greg have?"

So in one day I went from never hearing of diabetes to being the school expert. Now I know more about it than anyone else, even the teachers.

I know that it has something to do with the way your body uses food and that no one can catch it from you. I know it means you have to take shots of something called insulin, and you have to check your blood with a thing that looks like a pocket calculator. You have to eat healthy stuff, too.

And one more thing Mom and Dad told me about, something called an insulin reaction. They said if Greg didn't seem to be talking right, he might be having an insulin reaction and we should give him something sweet, like orange juice.

I think that's funny. He isn't supposed to have anything sweet, but that's what we give him if he has an insulin reaction. If you're wondering why, it's because a reaction means he has too much insulin and he needs something to use it up.

Anyway, all that worried me. And when Mom and Dad brought Greg home a few days later, he looked thin and kind of sad, so I tried to cheer him up with our "high five" sign. But he barely did it with me.

He only smiled a little and said, "How's it going, Squirt?" He gave me a punch on the arm, too, but it didn't feel right.

After Greg came home from the hospital, he stopped going to basketball practice or lifting weights. I was going to ask him about it when we went to bed—we usually talk after we put the light out— but he pretended to be asleep.

So little by little, I began to feel like I was *his* big brother, like I had to take care of him now instead of him taking care of me.

But I knew Greg would feel bad if I told him that. He hadn't even wanted me to help him back on the bike that time. So I didn't say anything.

Friday after school I went into the schoolyard. I thought about the times I had watched Greg shoot baskets there, and I felt awful.

Things went on like that for a couple more weeks. Then everything blew up.

In a way, it happened because I'm so short. I was sitting in the front row—where else?—in homeroom, and a note came in from the principal. It said that because Yardine Wright had moved away, there would be a meeting in Room 120 to fill her place on the Student Council. They wanted a representative from each homeroom.

Miss Albert just looked up, saw me, and said, "Danny, you go."

Sometimes it's good to sit in the front row. Only this

time, it wasn't, because after they got all us representatives together in Room 120, Adele said we should just elect Greg.

Everyone started shouting, "Yeh, Greg. We want Greg," and stuff like that, but Miss Shank said, "We have to use parliamentary procedure. Greg has been nominated. Now, does anyone have anything to say about him?"

Adele started yakking about how he knew everyone in school and what a good job he'd do. But my stomach was tightening like someone had hit it—I had a problem, the kind I would have told Greg about, once.

Finally I blurted out, "I don't think you should vote for my brother."

You'd have thought I nuked the place. "I don't think he wants to be on the Student Council," I added. Then I finished it off. "He won't accept."

Miss Shanks said, "Well, you're his brother so I guess you know. We don't want to have to meet again, so we'll pick someone else." To make it worse, you know who they picked? That jerk who took my apple that time, Billy Frazer.

I should have known Greg would find out, but I never guessed how fast. It was like he was bugging the meeting. I think Adele went right out and told him. She said I was jealous.

But I wasn't jealous. That wasn't it at all. I did it because I thought Greg was sick. I wanted to take care of him. I thought if he took the Student Council job he might get sicker with all the meetings and everything. Hey, it isn't easy being a good brother when everything changes so fast.

Anyway, Greg was sitting on his bed when I came

home that day. I knew it was going to be awful. I was right. His face got red when I walked in, and he shouted, "You crud! You're really something! I never knew you could sink so low."

But I couldn't tell him what I was really thinking. In a funny way, I knew it was better if he was mad at me than if I said I was taking care of him.

Dinner was awful that night. Greg didn't look at me at all. It wasn't the funny kind of not looking at you, like the time he told Mom to tell me to pass the bread, and I told Mom to tell him he could get the bread himself, and we both burst out laughing. This time, he was really angry!

It was hard to take, him being angry, and me not being able to tell him why, but still worrying about his diabetes. The next day I didn't feel like going home. I just went to the schoolyard again. I thought there might be a basketball practice.

But it wasn't the team practicing. It was Greg shooting baskets by himself. I couldn't understand. I thought he was sick. He didn't know I was there until he turned around.

"You spying on me, Danny?" he shouted.

"No."

I walked up to him slowly. "Can I talk to you a minute, Greg?"

"What do you want?" He walked away a little, dribbling the ball.

"Greg, I thought you couldn't shoot baskets anymore."

"Why not?"

"On account of the diabetes."

"What does diabetes have to do with shooting baskets?"

"Well, you stopped going to practice. You stopped lifting weights and all that."

Greg shook his head. "That's cause they were getting me stabilized on the right amount of insulin. Once they know how my body is doing, I can get back into sports. I told Coach Jacobs I have to check my blood at half-time, and he just said, 'No problem.' "

"So you could have been on the Student Council?"

"Of course."

"Greg, that's why I told them not to vote for you. I was worried about you."

He stopped dribbling the ball and looked at me. "You nut! You thought I couldn't be on the Student Council because of my diabetes?"

"Yeh. Something like that."

He shook his head like he couldn't believe it. Then he gave me a little punch on the arm, and this time it felt right. "Guess it's been hard on you, too, kid, me getting diabetes."

All at once he threw the ball right at me. I dribbled, jumped, aimed at the hoop, and missed. When I got the rebound, Greg picked me up, ran with me to the basket, and let me drop it clean in.

Like I said, the best thing about me is my brother, Greg.

Only now I think he thinks that maybe one of the best things about him is me.

Diabetes is New to Me

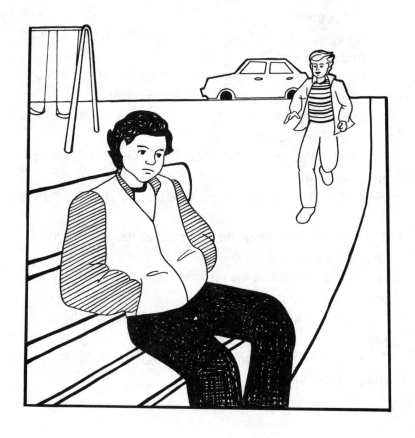

The Lie

by Marcia Levine Mazur

"Did you ever tell a lie?" Debbie asked her best friend, Erica. The girls were on their way home from school, but Debbie might just as well have stayed home that Tuesday. She hadn't heard anything the teacher had said. She was thinking about the lie.

"Who did you lie to?" Erica asked.

"My mom and dad."

"But why?"

"Never mind." Suddenly Debbie didn't want to tell Erica. Erica didn't have diabetes. How could she understand?

Besides, she wished it would all go away—the glucose meter, the doctor, most of all, the lie. But she couldn't stop thinking about it.

After supper, when she sat in the living room pretending to do homework, she was really thinking about how she could explain to Mom and Dad.

When they came into the room, Debbie even started to tell them. "Mom, Dad . . . "

"What is it, honey?"

She stopped talking. They trusted her. They thought she was so grown up. How could she tell them she had lied? "Oh, nothing," she answered, and just turned a page as if she were reading.

"Tell Dad what Dr. Bloom said this morning, Deb," Mom asked.

Debbie took a deep breath. "Well," she began, "he said something was wrong with my blood glucose records."

"What?" her father asked.

"They're just not right," Debbie answered slowly.

"How does he know?"

Why wouldn't Dad just drop it?

Debbie shrugged her shoulders. "Oh, just because he took some more tests. He said my notebook numbers didn't fit with his tests."

Her mother finished the story for her. "Dr. Bloom said Debbie could have gotten sick, because we didn't know her real blood glucose readings."

Mom and Dad went back into the kitchen. Debbie tried to hear what they were saying. She could tell that Dad was angry.

"I'm going to write a letter to the company that makes that glucose meter." He pounded on the kitchen table. "It shouldn't have broken in three months."

Debbie was scared. She knew the glucose meter wasn't broken. They only thought it was broken because she had lied.

They had bought it to help her do her glucose checks. And now they were going to march into that store and tell everyone there that it was broken. The man in the store would show them that it wasn't broken, and they would know she had been lying.

Several weeks earlier, Debbie had stopped doing her blood checks. She started putting down the same numbers she had gotten the week before. And she just kept doing it.

Now Debbie scrunched up her toes inside her sneakers. Why did they have to go and buy that dumb glucose meter anyway?

Of course, it had been her own fault. She had asked them to buy it. She said it would help her do her blood checks. And when she opened the box, she was so excited. And Mom and Dad were excited, too.

Then one day she told them she could do all her own glucose checks herself without anyone watching.

At first Mom had said, "I'm not sure, Deb. That's a lot to do by yourself."

"But, Mom," Debbie answered, "you always tell me how grown up I am." So they had said she could take her own glucose checks. Then Dad had bought her a blue notebook to write the numbers in.

At first it had been such a good feeling. She had taken her glucose readings every day and had always written the numbers in the notebook.

But after a couple of weeks, it wasn't so exciting anymore. And sometimes Erica was waiting for her to jump rope, or there was the after-school TV special. Or she was just tired of doing those checks.

That's when she had started putting the same numbers down every day.

What made it worse was that every time Mom asked her, "Deb, did you check your glucose?" she'd always answered, "Sure."

Right from the start, she had wanted to tell them. One night after dinner she took a deep breath and almost started to explain. Suddenly Mom had come over and hugged her. "We're so proud of you, Debbie, taking care of yourself so well."

And she couldn't tell. In fact, that made her feel so bad she'd started checking again. But it didn't last. She went back to copying the old numbers again. She was so sure no one would ever find out.

Until the day when Dr. Bloom had told Mom and Dad

the numbers didn't fit.

And now Mom and Dad thought the glucose meter was broken.

Finally, Dad came out of the kitchen with her bedtime snack. But even after she was in bed, Debbie couldn't sleep. Telling a lie, she learned, keeps you awake.

The next morning Erica asked her what she had lied about.

She told her. "My blood glucose checks. I told Mom and Dad that I always check my blood glucose. But I don't."

"Why did you do that?"

"You would too, if you had to prick your finger and do a blood glucose check a couple of times every day."

"What's it like, doing a glucose check?" Erica asked.

"I'll show you," Debbie answered.

After school, when they got to the house, Debbie took Erica to her room. Erica picked up the glucose meter. "What's this?"

"That's the glucose meter."

"Let me watch."

"You really want to?"

"Oh, yes."

Debbie took a drop of blood from her own finger.

"You have to do that every time?" Erica could hardly believe it.

"Yep." Debbie told her. "You have to get the blood to check."

"You're pretty brave, Deb. I couldn't do that every day."

Debbie looked at Erica, but didn't say anything. Debbie never thought she'd like anyone to watch her do

her blood glucose check. But it was kind of nice to have
Erica say she was brave.

"Now I have to write it in this little book," she
explained. She took a pencil and wrote down the number.

"I think that's neat," Erica said.

"But how would you like to do it all the time?"

"That would be tough. Is that why you lied and just
wrote down the numbers?"

"I guess so," Debbie answered.

"But why don't you just tell what happened?"

"I want to, Erica . . . I just can't."

Just then Debbie's mother called, "Girls, would you
come out here now? "

Mrs. Stanley was standing at the front door with her
coat on. "Deb, I want you to come with me. We're meeting
Dad at the store. We're going to return that glucose meter.
I'm very angry about it."

Erica looked at Debbie and shrugged her shoulders as
if to say "I'm sorry." Then she left.

Debbie put her coat on slowly and walked outside with
her mother.

"Mom," she said.

"What is it?"

"Could we go back into the house?"

"Did you forget something?"

"Sort of."

They went back in, and Debbie sat down on the couch.

"I forgot to tell you the truth."

"What do you mean?"

"Mom, there's nothing wrong with the glucose meter.
There's something wrong with me."

"Are you sick?"

"No. I mean I lied."

"About what?"

"About checking my blood glucose all the time."

"Didn't you do it?"

"No, I just wrote the old numbers down again."

"But why didn't you tell us?"

"Because you were so proud of me. And you trusted me. And you were so happy I was doing it myself. I didn't want to make you mad. You said I was such a big girl."

Mrs. Stanley sat down next to Debbie and put her arms around her.

"Oh, Debbie. We just didn't realize. Dad and I acted like you were 20 years old or something. I thought that if I was just somewhere in the house when you were checking your blood, that was enough."

"Mom, I'm sorry. I didn't mean to be bad."

"You're not bad, Debbie. It's tough having diabetes and going to school and wanting to play and trying out for the team and doing homework. It's rough having to do blood glucose checks, too.

"Besides, Debbie," her mother smiled. "Dad and I have a secret, too."

"You do? What?"

"We're glad you still want us to help you with your diabetes. We were sad when we thought you didn't need us anymore."

Debbie snuggled up to her mother and hugged her tight. Her mother hugged back. "You know, Debbie, mothers and fathers like to feel they're still needed, even though their children are growing up."

Stay Away From Me

by Marcia Levine Mazur

"Where in the world is Carlos?" Joseph thought. He was so busy wondering about Carlos, he hardly noticed the nurse setting the glucose meter beside his bed.

"You're doing great," she told him, but Joseph knew she was only trying to cheer him up. Not that he didn't need cheering. It isn't easy to learn you have diabetes.

But it was Carlos, not the diabetes, who was on his mind right now. "My so-called best friend," Joseph thought, "my best friend who hasn't even visited me in the hospital."

Joseph's class had sent a huge greeting card. "We miss you!!!!" was spread across the front. That had to be Mary Lyons. And, "Hey, Joe, I know you're lazy, but this is ridiculous." Only Larry Crane would have written that. All the lines were funny, but there was no line at all from Carlos.

"Where is he?" Joseph wondered again. "He should have visited me," Joseph told himself, "especially with the zoo thing going on."

Although the zoo thing was their best adventure yet, Joseph and Carlos had first become friends at basketball practice. Joseph had noticed Carlos missing baskets, so he'd stepped in and showed Carlos how to arc the ball so it went through the hoop instead of missing and bouncing off the backboard.

Later, when Joseph got a "D" in English, Carlos taught him all about verbs and adverbs and pronouns.

But the best thing they had done together was the zoo thing. Joseph had just started thinking about it when Mom rushed into his hospital room, kissed him, and plopped onto the chair next to the bed.

"How you doing?" Dad was right behind her.

"I'm fine," he told them in a quiet voice, "I'm just fine."

"You don't sound it." Mom said.

She was a little too light-hearted, Joseph thought. Just like the nurse, he knew she was trying to cheer him up.

"Books, papers, candy, gifts." A voice sang through the door and Joseph waved to Sarah, the gift-cart lady. "Want anything?" she asked.

"No," Dad answered.

"Wait. You have the paper?" Joseph asked.

"Sure."

Sarah handed the evening paper to Joseph, who slipped it under his pillow while Dad paid for it.

"Well, that's something new," Dad said. "An interest in the news."

But it wasn't the news Joseph wanted to see.

He waited until Mom and Dad had left, then pulled out the paper. It made a rustling sound as he tossed the front section to the end of the bed and took out the "What's Happening" part.

A minute later he threw that to the end of the bed too. Joseph had thought the contest was over today, but now he saw that it wouldn't end till tomorrow. The ad said, "LAST DAY TO NAME THE BABY ELEPHANT. GIVE THE ZOO'S NEW BABY GIRL A NAME AND WIN $150."

He would have to wait another day to find out who

won. Not that it mattered. He and Carlos would never split the prize now.

Only a week ago Carlos had come running up with the paper. "Look Joe-Joe (Carlos was the only one who got away with calling him Joe-Joe), one hundred fifty dollars! And all we have to do is name the baby elephant."

Joseph whistled. "What would we do with the money?"

"Take our families to dinner together, of course," Carlos answered.

Although Joseph and Carlos never talked about it, they both knew their families were different from each other. Carlos' parents, the Garcias, had been born in Mexico. Joseph's family, the Walters, had come from England a long time ago. But every family member of his that Joseph knew had been born in the United States.

Somehow, the boys had never invited their families anywhere together.

"When we win the contest we'll all go to a big fancy restaurant," Carlos said. Joseph saw that Carlos was really excited. "And you and I will pay for it, and our parents will get to know each other."

"But how will we know what to name the elephant?"

"I got that figured out, too," Carlos announced. "We're going to ride our bikes to the zoo Saturday and look at her. Once we see her, we'll know."

After Carlos said it, Joseph was sure it would work. And early Saturday morning he called to Mom and Dad, "Going bike riding with Carlos!"

"Be back by noon," Mom answered.

"OK."

Joseph didn't know it then, but he would be back much

later than noon.

He hopped on his bike, met Carlos at the corner, and the two began pedaling at top speed. But after a few minutes, Joseph felt funny and had to stop in the park to take a drink. Then he had to go to the bathroom.

At the zoo, he had to take more drinks and go to the bathroom again. "You OK?" Carlos asked.

"Sure. Just real thirsty."

But when they finally got a look at the baby elephant, they forgot everything else.

"Boy is she cute!" Joseph just stared. He thought she looked like a toy, one that could move, and toss her trunk, and follow her great big mother around. "She's really something," he whispered to Carlos. "What should we name her?"

"Linda," Carlos answered. "That's Spanish for beautiful."

"Linda. Yeh. I like that. Linda."

Carlos and Joseph started back, proud of themselves. They had carried out their plan—visited the zoo, and surely picked the winning name.

But when they were almost home, Joseph fell off his bike. Then the road began to look blurry to him. Home late, it took him 15 minutes to explain what had happened.

Lying in the hospital now, he remembered that zoo day. It had been the day all this diabetes stuff had started.

Joseph hadn't felt well the rest of the day, and Carlos had filled out the entry form, wrote in the name they had chosen—Linda—and sent it to the paper.

The next day Joseph went to the doctor and then to the hospital. He didn't hear from Carlos again.

Saturday, four days after Joseph went into the hospital,

the doctor said he could go home. Mom was all excited.

Back home, she pointed to a drawer in the kitchen. "This is for your diabetes things," she told him. "No one else will touch it."

Early Monday morning, Joseph took off for school. He wanted to be in his seat when everyone came in. That way he wouldn't have to answer questions, or say hello to Carlos.

No one made a big fuss, and he was glad of that. Colleen, Rob, and Steve just said, "Hi. Great to have you back." And Miss Rickoff welcomed him before she started class.

Carlos came in late, his head bent low so he didn't have to see anyone.

Every hour or so, Joseph glanced at Carlos. But Carlos never seemed to be paying attention to the lesson. "What's his problem?" Joseph thought. "He doesn't have diabetes."

As soon as the final bell rang, Joseph shot out of school. He didn't want to talk to anyone, certainly not to Carlos. At home, he scrunched down on the couch until he heard the delivery boy slap the afternoon paper against the door.

Then he grabbed it and turned again to the "What's Happening" section. "ANNOUNCING THE WINNER OF THE 'NAME THE BABY ELEPHANT CONTEST.' SAY 'HELLO' TO BABY HENRIETTA."

"Henrietta!!" Joseph threw the paper onto the couch. "Henrietta! What a name for an elephant!"

He slouched into his room. No sir! He was never going to make friends, or enter another contest again, even if he could win a hundred million dollars.

As soon as dinner was over, Joseph scurried back to

his room. Although he had a barrelful of homework, he lay down with his clothes on, snapped on the radio, and pulled the covers over his head.

A few hours later Dad came in with crackers and milk. The nurse had brought him the same thing in the hospital and Joseph knew he had to have a snack because of the diabetes. But he was hungry anyway.

"You've been having a tough time, haven't you?" Dad asked, and Joseph nodded. He was glad Dad didn't say anything about homework.

Joseph fell asleep almost as soon as Dad left the room. But he sat up when the phone rang. He was surprised to see how dark it was outside.

"Carlos?" He heard Dad say. "Why, no. He's not here. Wait. I'll check."

He heard a knock on his door. "Joseph, do you know where Carlos is? He took off just before dinner and his parents don't know where he is."

"No," Joseph called.

He didn't know exactly where Carlos was, but he knew exactly what had happened.

Carlos had looked at the paper too. And he had also been angry that they hadn't won. But why had Carlos taken off? After all, it wasn't like it cost money to get into the contest. And nobody even knew they had entered it.

Their name, "Linda," had been Carlos' idea, of course. He had said it meant beautiful in Spanish. But why should he get so upset if it didn't win?

Suddenly Joseph rushed out of his room pulling his jacket on. "I think I know where Carlos is," he called. "He's in the schoolyard, at the basketball court."

He and Dad hurried out. "I'm coming too," Mom

called, rushing after them.

The minute Dad pulled up to the dark court, Joseph jumped out. It was chilly, but he didn't notice because he saw Carlos sitting on the bench alone in the dark.

Joseph hurried to the bench. "Hey, what's wrong? We were worried."

"They didn't pick my name," Carlos answered, as if he and Joseph had been talking for weeks.

"Yeh. I know. So what?"

"You don't know? They didn't pick it because it's Spanish."

"Spanish? What does that have to do with it?"

"They don't like Spanish names. Only American names."

"I know it's American," Joseph told him. "And it's not nearly as good as Linda. But I don't think they even knew Linda was Spanish. I didn't know. Maybe the zoo keeper's mother is named Henrietta or something."

Carlos laughed at that. Then suddenly, he jumped up and moved away.

"Where are you going?" Joseph asked.

"I'm sorry, Joe-Joe. I don't care about myself, but I have three little sisters, and my mother gets sick very easy. Last year I had the flu and all of them caught it from me. I can't let them catch diabetes. I was going to write you a letter and send you all the money from the contest."

"You idiot," Joseph said. "You can't catch diabetes. It's like having a broken leg. You just can't catch it. Boy, for a guy who gets A's in English, you sure don't know much about diabetes."

Of course, Joseph didn't tell Carlos that he had asked the doctor the same question.

Carlos looked surprised. "No kidding, Joe-Joe? You can't catch it?"

"No kidding."

Carlos started to laugh again.

"Race you to the car," Joseph said.

The boys ran, panting, across the dark school yard, but even before they noticed who won, they saw that Carlos' mother and father had driven up, too.

"I thought you'd be here," Carlos' mother said. Then she hugged her son hard. "Don't you ever do that again," she said between hugs.

"Why don't we all go get a yogurt or something?" Mrs. Walters said. "There's an all-night grocery on the corner."

The two families parked next to each other, and all of them walked into the store together. Carlos' mother was still holding onto his shoulder as if she might lose him again.

Everyone ordered fat-free frozen yogurts and stood at the counter slurping and talking. Joseph poked Carlos in the ribs, "Big fine restaurant, huh?" he said, reminding Carlos of how they were going to spend their prize money.

"Well, at least we got them together," Carlos answered.

"Say." Mrs. Walters turned to Mrs. Garcia. "Would you like to help with the PTA's next fund raiser?"

"I'd love to," Mrs. Garcia answered.

"Great. I'll give you the president's number. She's very friendly. Just ask for Henrietta."

Neither the Garcias nor the Walters understood why their sons burst out laughing so hard they dropped down and rolled on the floor.

The Big, Bad Bikers

by Marcia Levine Mazur

Like most 11-year olds, Bobby Jensen had a special hero. But his hero wasn't someone his friends would choose. They all wanted to be football stars like Jonathan Hayes, or basketball players like Michael Jordan. Not Bobby.

Some of the girls in his class wanted to be Olympic ice skaters. Not Bobby.

No. He wanted to be like Greg LeMond, the world champion bicycle rider. Bobby decided he wanted to be like Greg LeMond the day he saw the Tour De France bicycle race on TV. He could almost feel the excitement through the screen when Greg shot across the finish line, his hands raised in victory.

Of course, he let his mom and dad know his new dream—to own a bicycle. And although they said, "We'll see," seven months later, on his 12th birthday, Bobby got his sleek thin-tired bicycle. It was black with yellow tiger stripes and glistening silver handlebars. He also got a black helmet.

Bobby loved to jump up onto the seat of his bicycle, slide his feet onto the pedals and take off, his face chilled by the breeze from his own speed.

Yet some days it all didn't feel right.

One time it was because he had a headache, another day the trees looked kind of fuzzy even before his foot hit the pedal. On top of that, he was losing weight.

Something was wrong.

Then Mr. Jensen decided Bobby needed to join a

155

bicycle club. But when Mr. Jensen called the sports center, they told him there were no bicycle clubs. So he called the Department of Parks. But they said the city had no place for such a club to practice.

"I beg your pardon," Bobby's dad answered. "There's the bicycle track in the park by the zoo. If you let the club practice there, I'll be the coach."

The Department of Parks agreed.

Four boys and three girls signed up just on the first day. But none rode as fast as Bobby, except for a new boy on the next street, Chan Lee.

Mr. Jensen announced one club rule. "No one rides without a helmet."

Bobby was happiest when he and Chan were riding along the bike path. Chan and his mother had just moved to Bobby's California neighborhood, and Bobby and Chan would ride together for hours.

But Bobby wanted more.

That's why his heart started pounding the evening his father told him that another club had challenged them to a race. It was the Hamilton School Bike Club. They wore bright red tee-shirts that said "Hamilton's Heroes."

Mr. Jensen didn't waste time. "Let's make the challenge a relay race. Seven riders from each club. Each rider takes three turns around the track."

Everyone voted "yes" for the race, but they knew they had only one chance to win—Bobby.

They sent their challenge to the Hamilton Heroes, and the answer came back "It will be a pleasure to make you eat our dust," it said. Then in big red letters, "We are the Hamilton Heroes."

"Wow!" Chan spoke for all of them. Then he added,

"This will be my first race in this country. It will make my mother so proud if we win."

"We'll win," Bobby told him. "And the race will make us into a real club!" Mr. Jensen smiled at his son. The club had been meeting at different member's houses, and Mr. Jensen was always there because he was the coach.

"Let's get tee-shirts, too." Vic jumped up from his chair, "Yellow and orange ones."

"Good idea," Mr. Jensen nodded. "Does anyone have a club name?" Bobby whispered it through his teeth, "Big Bad Bikers."

"Yeh!!! Big Bad Bikers," everyone shouted it, until it became a sing-song. "We don't care if you like hikers. We're the club of Big Bad Bikers."

Mr. Jensen and the Hamilton coach set the race date two months away, Saturday, 2:00 P.M. And they got the Department of Parks to close off the track that afternoon so no one else would be on it.

It was clear that everyone in the club was excited. But to Bobby it was his first chance to roll across the finish line, shooting his hands over his head in victory, the way Greg LeMond did.

To Chan it was a chance to make his mother proud of his new American club.

But Bobby still wasn't feeling well. He hoped it was just the excitement, but he knew excitement didn't make you lose weight and get so thirsty that a gallon of water didn't help.

Then one night Bobby Jensen, hero of the Big Bad Bikers, wet the bed. He couldn't believe it. He didn't want his mom or dad to know, but Mrs. Jensen found out when she did the laundry, and instead of laughing or getting angry, she made a doctor's appointment for him.

Everything happened fast after that, the way trees whiz by in a race. Dr. Bloom put Bobby in the hospital and told him he had something Bobby thought sounded like a vegetable, diabetes. A nurse showed him how to give himself insulin shots.

But after she left each time, Bobby turned his face to the wall. He felt like his body was no longer his friend. He had practiced riding, he had worked hard, trained, and what for? Now he had a sickness he would never get rid of.

The Big Bad Bikers visited him in the hospital. The yellow and black tee-shirts had arrived, and they handed Bobby his, but when they left, he threw it into a corner.

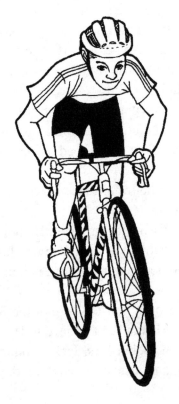

Why couldn't they understand? Now he had to learn about blood sugar and insulin and meal plans. How could he be a great biker?

Bobby was out of the hospital in a few days, but he didn't go near the bike track. Dr. Bloom told him he could ride as long as he and his family made sure his blood glucose was in good control. But Bobby didn't think a body that needed shots and a meal plan could ever win a race.

"Hey," his dad said, "You're feeling sorry for yourself. Get your diabetes under control and get back onto the track."

"Yeh? What am I supposed to do, stop before the finish line and check my blood glucose?"

Bobby felt hurt. No one understood. Even his own parents didn't understand. He rode alone the next few weeks.

Then the evening before the race Chan knocked quietly at the Jensen door. "Please, Bobby, come out and ride with me. I want the club to win, but I'm so nervous. We always rode together."

"Go away."

"Do it," his mom said. "Your sugar is in good control. The doctor said you could ride. So, go on."

"Oh, what the heck. Sure, I'll go."

Bobby and Chan rode around and around the neighborhood without talking. When a light breeze whipped up, Bobby said, "Let's stop."

But he didn't say it soon enough. Chan's tire caught in a hole, and he fell on his left leg. Bobby pulled Chan free, but the leg was bleeding. "Hey," Bobby told him softly, "You won't be riding that race tomorrow."

"What do you care? You won't even wear our tee-shirt." Chan looked away.

Bobby got his dad, and they took Chan to the emergency room.

The hospital halls were hushed. Mrs. Lee and Mr. Jensen were in the emergency room with Chan. The Big Bad Bikers sat in the empty waiting room. Finally, Vic said what everyone was thinking. "Why don't we just end the club? Without Bobby or Chan we'll never win that race."

"What are you talking about?" Bobby couldn't believe what he was hearing.

"You have nothing to say about it," Vic answered. "You won't even put on the tee-shirt."

"Heck," Danny nodded. "You're not even a Big Bad Biker. That diabetes is the biker." Danny looked around at his joke and they all laughed quietly.

"I think Danny's right," Tommy added. "That diabetes is riding you."

"You don't understand."

"Oh, we understand," Tommy said. "Your doctor said you could ride. But you won't even try."

One by one, as if it were planned, they peeled off their tee-shirts.

"What are you doing?" Bobby stood up and looked at them.

"We don't want to make fools of ourselves tomorrow." Danny said.

"So you're going to give up?" Bobby asked.

"Why not? You did," Vic threw at him. It was quiet then because someone had finally said it.

Bobby was confused. Didn't his friends see him the way he saw himself—poor Bobby, the kid with this sickness?

He started to walk away when someone—he never knew who—said softly, "And you don't even care about Chan."

"What?"

"You haven't thought how much he wants to make his mother proud of his new American club. That's why he was practicing."

Bobby suddenly realized that he hadn't thought about Chan—or anyone else—since he was diagnosed. He had only thought about his diabetes.

Chan came hobbling out of the emergency room. "Chan will be OK in a few days," his dad told the club, "but he won't be riding for awhile."

Bobby looked at Chan, but his friend turned his head away. Then Bobby grabbed the tee-shirt Vic had taken off, and pulled it right over his own shirt.

He walked over to the nurse's desk. "Can I see Dr. Bloom, please?"

"I'm sorry. He's gone home."

"Please, may I have his home number?"

"I can't give that out."

"This is an emergency."

The nurse looked at Bobby, then at the other club members. Finally, she nodded. "573-2100."

Bobby asked his father for a quarter to make the phone call. "Dr. Bloom, I'm really sorry to bother you like this, but this is Bobby Jensen and I want to know how to make sure I'm in good shape to ride in a bike race tomorrow."

The race started right at 2 o'clock. Most of the parents were there. A lot of other kids and even strangers were standing around the side of the track. Many cheered the Hamilton Heroes who whipped along as if a ghost were chasing them. They were winning from the beginning. At the end of the fourth group of riders, they were still ahead. "Eat our dust," one of them called.

Bobby was the last Big Bad Biker to ride. He waited, half sitting on the bike, one foot ready to hit the pedal and go, when Chan hobbled up. "Thanks Bobby. I knew you'd get back in the driver's seat."

Then it was time! Bobby jumped onto the seat, slapped the pedal down with his foot, and shot out on the black and yellow bicycle.

The Big Bad Bikers were a length behind, and Bobby pedaled as if he were Greg LeMond at the Tour de France, as if the whole world were watching, cheering him on. But after two times around the track he still hadn't caught up.

On his last lap Bobby was breathing hard, his feet pedaling like robots. But he was going faster and faster. In fact, he was going faster than ever. His body hadn't let him down! He could still be a champion.

He pedaled with all his heart, thinking about his good friend Chan. He pedaled faster and faster thinking about all the kids in the club. He pedaled for his mom and dad, and he pedaled for himself.

When the last Hamilton Hero rider looked back, he saw Bobby Jensen coming up on his right, passing, and whizzing across the finish line first, his hands raised high in the air in victory.

Sometimes You Need
A Little Magic

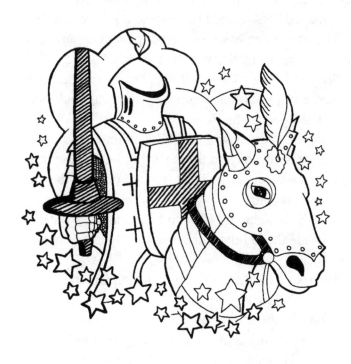

The Magic Tournament

by Marcia Levine Mazur

Dulcie had an odd feeling. She looked around the King Arthur exhibit in the museum and realized what it was. She was alone. No one else was there. The knights in their silvery armor, the ladies in long filmy dresses and cone-shaped hats seemed to be standing there just for her.

The class must have wandered to another part of the museum, she decided. Even the guard was gone.

So, just to see what it felt like, Dulcie reached out and touched a suit of armor. But before she could pull her hand back, it clanged to the floor.

"Oh, no! What have I done?" she thought.

She stooped down to lift the armor back into place, but couldn't resist fitting her hand into the palm of the knight's metal glove.

Did she imagine it? His hand was closing over hers! From inside the helmet came a voice, "Please take me home."

The room seemed to shake then, and Dulcie fell to the floor, too. She looked around for help.

Suddenly there were no walls or ceiling or floor. There was only open sky, and a knight sitting next to her in an open field. Had she gone home with him—back to the Middle Ages?

Quickly the knight pulled his helmet off, and they looked at each other. Why, he didn't look much older than she was!

"Who are you?" he asked. "How did you get here, and

why are you wearing men's pants?"

She wondered how she could understand him. Did time travel make you smart? "I'm Dulcie," she answered, "and I don't know how I got here, and these are girl's jeans."

Looking down at them, she decided time travel must make you dusty as well as smart. She stood and brushed herself off. "Where am I?"

"Why, you're in Darbytown, of course. On market day."

About half a mile away Dulcie saw a row of small stands, each with a yellow straw roof or brightly colored awning. Everywhere men and women were shouting; they all seemed to be selling things. Animals and children were racing in and out of the stands. They stood out against the green grass and the blue sky and she couldn't wait to get there.

She turned back to the knight. "And who are you?"

"I'll tell you if you help me stand up. This armor is heavy."

"OK," Dulcie said. "I'll try something my brother taught me." With the knight lying flat on his back, knees bent, she stood on top of his toes, held his hands, and pulled. He bounced to his feet. and the two of them burst out laughing.

"Now, who are you?" she asked.

The knight put his helmet under his arm and announced seriously, "I am Cedric, second son of Sir Darby of Darbyshire."

He made a sweep with his hands. "And these were once my father's lands."

"Why doesn't he own them now?"

"He lost them in a joust to Chadwick the Unsettled."

"A joust?"

"Yes, a battle where two knights on horseback try to unseat each other with long lances."

"But how did your father lose his lands?"

"There is a decree in this valley that a knight may challenge a knight-landowner to a joust. If the knight wins, he takes the lands. But the landowner may win them back within three years."

"So, Chadwick won your father's lands fairly?" she asked.

"No! Chadwick jabbed my father's horse. It jumped and my father fell."

Dulcie shook her head.

Cedric looked away from her, but kept talking. "And now three years are nearly over and I must win tomorrow's joust, or our lands will be gone forever. If only. . . ."

"If only?" Dulcie asked. She wanted him to keep talking.

"If only my older brother, Richard, were alive. He was a real knight."

"But you are a real knight."

"No," Cedric spoke softly. "I am the second son. Only Richard was trained for knighthood."

"What happened to Richard?"

"It's so sad, Dulcie. He had the wasting sickness. First he weakened, and then he asked for water, water all the time. For two years he wasted away, and then he died."

Dulcie remembered when she, too, had asked for water. But she had seen a doctor, and she was doing fine now.

"Perhaps the wasting sickness is what we call diabetes,"

she said softly.

"Do you, too, know someone with this sickness?"

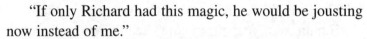

"Yes. Me! But I also know a magic liquid that lets people with the wasting sickness do anything they want.

"A magic liquid?"

"Sure. Insulin."

"If only Richard had this magic, he would be jousting now instead of me."

Dulcie said nothing, and together they walked to the booths. Even from a distance, Dulcie found the smells overpowering. They came from the mounds of strange foods, and from fat dripping into the fire from a roasting pig, and from other meats sputtering loudly as they cooked.

"I have come to buy a steed for tomorrow's joust," Cedric said, "But I have only a few coins."

"Hey, I'll buy you a steed, I mean a horse!" Dulcie told him as they walked.

"You? But why?"

"Because I want you to win your lands back. And, besides, it will be fun."

They walked into a stable where an old man was playing music on a stick with holes in it. People were bargaining loudly. The smell was awful. Horses were snorting and stamping the ground, and huge black flies were buzzing everywhere.

Cedric pointed to a sleek black horse with a white patch around one eye. "That is the one."

Dulcie looked at the horse's owner. Will you take this for that steed?" she asked. Then she reached into her waist carryall, pushed the "play" button on her tape player, and watched his face as rock music blasted out.

Instantly. the crowd pulled back. Some screamed, others ran. One woman yelled, "Devil! Witch!"

Even Cedric looked terrified. "Have you indeed come from the Devil?"

"No," she laughed. "Hey, even some people in my time don't like this."

"Your time? When's that?"

"I'm from the future, hundreds of years from now."

"Hundreds of years from now? I can't believe there'll be such wonderful things then."

"But there will be, Cedric. There will be."

She handed the tape player to the horse owner who took it eagerly.

Quietly Cedric and Dulcie led the horse out. "Let's call him Sir Lancelot," Dulcie said, as Cedric helped her climb on. Then, with Cedric walking and Dulcie riding Sir Lancelot, they left the Darbytown market.

About two hours later they rounded a curve and Cedric stopped. "Yon is Darby Castle, readying for the tournament." The castle stood high on a hill. To Dulcie, the turrets seemed to touch the sky. Red and yellow flags flapped there in the wind.

There was a little stream of water circling the castle. Dulcie knew that was the moat.

The drawbridge over the moat was down, and men and women were shouting, balancing baskets on their heads, and pulling animals or carts over it, preparing for the tournament. It was loud and colorful and lively.

Cedric sighed and looked away. "I'll never be good enough to win our lands back," he said. Dulcie knew she just had to give him confidence.

They let Sir Lancelot graze before tethering him to a tree. Then both sat down, and Cedric fell asleep in his armor.

Not Dulcie. She injected her insulin and ate a mushy peanut butter sandwich. "Boy," she thought, "It's a good thing I was going to Shirley's after the museum. Otherwise I wouldn't have filled syringes in my carryall."

It was dark now, and she stared up at the stars. They must be the same ones she would see centuries later—if she ever got back home. Time was running out. Everyone would be worried, and she only had one more syringe of insulin left. She had to get back.

But first she had to find a way to make Cedric believe in himself. She fell asleep trying to think of something.

She awoke as the sun was rising, and laughed when Cedric couldn't stand in his armor again. She used the same trick and got him on his feet.

"You are as bright as the sun, Dulcie," he said. "I wish I could take your brightness into battle with me."

"That's it!" Dulcie called. "You can take it. You can take your own sun."

She opened her carryall and dug out her pen flashlight. "Here is a lamp that will make you more powerful than any other knight." To herself she thought, "Boy, I hope these batteries hold up."

Dulcie watched Cedric's eyes pop when she turned on the light. "Light without fire," he whispered. "You must live in a truly wondrous time."

"Yes," Dulcie said. "I guess I do live in a truly wondrous time. I just never thought about it that way before."

Carefully, as if it would burn him, Cedric took the flashlight, reached inside his armor, and put it near his heart.

And now, breakfast," Dulcie said. She injected herself with her last syringe.

"Ta da. . .," Dulcie held up the last peanut butter sandwich. "This is not magic, but you may like it." He did. Then Cedric found a patch of wild berries ready to be picked. Dulcie knew she should wash them before she ate, but, of course, these berries had never been sprayed.

Afterwards, Dulcie shined Cedric's armor with the bottom of her tee-shirt, and listened to the musicians playing as people gathered outside the castle.

The sun grew higher and men in bright colored suits— half purple, half yellow—came onto the top turrets of the castle, and blew on long shiny horns.

"It's time," Cedric told her.

"Are you afraid, Cedric?"

"Not anymore." He tapped the spot where the flashlight was.

Then Cedric put his hands on Dulcie's shoulders. "Now it is my turn to explain something. When a knight goes into battle, he carries his lady's favor. You know, a kerchief, a flower, a ribbon."

"But I have no ribbons," Dulcie answered. "No, wait! I do." She unclipped her museum I.D. badge that said 'Dulcie Kahn, John F. Kennedy School.' It had a red ribbon hanging from it. Cedric put it inside his armor next to the flashlight.

"And now," he said softly, "I must go on alone."

Dulcie helped him onto Sir Lancelot, then handed him

his lance. "Shall I see you again?" he asked.

"I think not, Cedric. I must return to my own world." She smiled up at him, her own knight in shining armor. "But how will I know if you've won?"

"I will have the musicians sound a gong three times, so loudly that you will hear it wherever you are. And now, I salute you." He tipped her shoulder with his lance.

She reached up to touch the spot, but someone's hand was there, shaking her.

"Dulcie, are you all right?" It was Ms. Davis, her teacher. "The armor fell down somehow. It must have hit you."

"What? Oh, yes. I'm fine. Fine." Dulcie stood and brushed the dust off her jeans. She almost cried, remembering the last time she had done that.

"But where is your I.D. badge dear?" Ms. Davis asked.

"My badge?" Dulcie touched the spot where her I.D. had been and smiled. Just then the clock on the guard's desk sounded three times.

"Don't worry, Ms. Davis. My badge is in a very safe place—with someone who has just won a great victory."

Riding the Woolly Mammoth!

by Marcia Levine Mazur

Connie stared at the huge animals behind the glass. She knew they weren't real. The museum just made them to show people how animals looked in prehistoric times.

But then, nothing in Connie's life seemed real anymore. Not since the doctor told her she had a disease with a funny-sounding name, diabetes.

All at once, she had to have insulin injections, eat carefully, and carry sugar in case she felt dizzy. That was about as unreal as you can get, she thought.

Even being in the natural history museum seemed unusual. Since when did Mom and Dad stay home from work and take her to a museum the minute she asked?

Ever since they learned she had diabetes, that's when.

Connie studied the animals behind the glass. Most of them looked like they wanted to charge across the museum floor.

Except the biggest. It looked a lot like an elephant, only much bigger, with lots of shaggy hair hanging from its sides, and whitish tusks so enormous they curved around and pointed upward. "Boy, I'd stay away from those," she thought.

But the funny thing was, the enormous animal seemed to be looking right at her, and it's eyes seemed so sad.

Connie stepped closer to the glass and whispered, "I know who you are. You're a woolly mammoth, and you lived thousands of years ago when the earth was covered with snow and ice. But why are you so unhappy?"

172

"Coming?" Mom's voice broke into Connie's day-dream. Mom and Dad were already at the next case, and Connie moved on to join them, waving good-bye to her new friend.

Afterward, in the museum shop, Connie announced that she wanted a stuffed woolly mammoth. Mom and Dad bought it without saying a word. Still totally unreal, Connie thought.

Back home they helped her check her blood glucose and take her insulin before they all sat down to eat. Then she just sat and watched television the rest of the evening, and no one told her to turn it off. "When is it going to get real again around here?" she thought.

A lot of the unreal stuff had started three weeks ago, after Dr. Gold had told them Connie had diabetes. Connie had cried, and Dr. Gold said, "You'll do fine, Connie. And remember, you can call me anytime you need me."

Then Mom had hugged her. "See, Connie, you're not alone. We are all here to help you."

Dad had come over and put his arms around her. "You can do it, Connie. You can take care of yourself. And when the going gets tough, you let us know."

And that was when the unreal stuff started, like buying her whatever she wanted and taking her anywhere she asked to go.

Connie yawned as soon as she got into bed. The trip to the museum had made her tired, and she fell asleep hold-ing the woolly mammoth. Only the mammoth seemed to grow bigger and bigger until she couldn't get her arm around it, so big that it filled the bed, so big that it would soon fill the room.

Quickly Connie and the mammoth got up and ran out

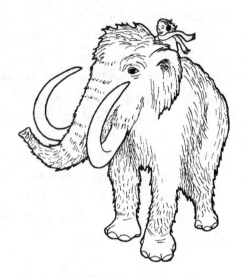

the front door. The mammoth was still small enough to get through.

They ran back to the museum, back behind the glass, back into the last Ice Age. Only this time, Connie was there, too.

The mammoth, now its full size, wrapped its long trunk around Connie's waist, lifted her way up, and settled her on its great back. She grabbed hold of its long hairs and held on tight.

Then she inched forward to the enormous ear and shouted, "What's your name?"

"I'm Dooley the Woolly," he said in a voice so deep it almost sounded like it was coming from thousands of years ago.

"Well, Dooley, why are you so sad?"

"I don't feel well. I'm so thirsty I could drink up all the snow in my Ice Age, but I don't know what's wrong."

Connie was pretty sure she knew. "If I only had Dr. Gold here," she thought.

And there he was, Dr. Gold, standing in front of them cleaning his glasses and shivering! He had the collar of his white coat turned up and icicles were hanging from his nose. "I'm freezing," he said. "I don't belong in any Ice Age."

"Then what are you doing here?" Connie asked, still surprised.

"You said you needed help and I said you could always call on me."

"Wow," she said. "Fantastic. Well Dooley here is sick. Do you know what's wrong with him?"

Dr. Gold seemed annoyed. "Of course I know. I've already given him some tests. Since he's a mammal, he has a pancreas, and it's obvious that it isn't working well. So I think he needs an insulin injection. Here, you give it to him."

He handed her an insulin syringe as large as a baseball bat, and disappeared. Only a big white snowball remained where Dr. Gold had been shivering in his white coat.

Connie tucked the syringe under her arm and looked at Dooley. "Now let's see," she said. "I usually get my injection in my arm, but you don't seem to have arms."

Dooley's head hung low. "I don't feel well," he said.

She made a quick decision. "Get me down to your leg. I guess that's the closest thing to an arm."

Carefully, Dooley curled his trunk around Connie's waist again. Then he slowly lowered her down his tall body to his front left leg.

Connie hung there, upside down, dizzy, her hair hanging in her face, trying to find a spot to give Dooley an injection.

It wasn't easy. The woolly mammoth had thick hair longer than her whole body. When she found her way through the hair, there seemed to be a blanket of wool growing underneath.

"I guess that's why they call them woolly," she thought.

Finally she brushed aside enough hair and wool to give Dooley an injection on his leg.

But as soon as she finished the injection, the huge syringe slipped and landed on the ground. "I wonder what they'll think of that if they dig it up in the twentieth century," she said, laughing to herself. "OK, now please lift me back up."

Dooley raised his trunk and swung her onto his back again.

"Whew," she said. "That was rough. OK. Now you have to eat something. That's so the insulin can have some food to work on," she explained.

Dooley lowered his head and started nibbling the bits of grass that grew just above the snow and ice. He nibbled and chewed and nibbled and chewed until finally he seemed full.

Then he started playfully tossing Connie up and down on his back.

"Hey, hold on," she yelled.

"Watch this," he said, and he started running. Connie clutched the hair on his back and bounced along laughing and singing "Old MacDonald Had A Farm" as loud as she could—until suddenly Dooley stopped. Instead of going forward, he began dropping down like an elevator.

"I'm stuck in a crevasse!" he shouted. "My uncle

Gooley got stuck in one last year and never got out."

"What's a crevasse?" Connie yelled.

"A split in the ice. My mother always told me to watch out for crevasses.

"Well, pull out, Dooley, pull out!" she shouted.

"I can't. I'm stuck."

"Oh, I wish Dad were here," Connie said to herself.

"Can I help?" Dad was standing a few feet away, wearing his heavy plaid jacket and bright red scarf. He was calmly attaching a chain to the back of a black pickup truck. "Now we'll fasten the other end around your friend here," he said.

"But, Dad, where did you come from?"

"You said you needed help and I told you I'd always be there if you needed me."

"Wow," was all Connie could say.

Dad was already climbing down the ice to get the chain around Dooley's huge body.

"Hurry! Hurry!" Connie cried.

Dad locked the chain around Dooley's middle, then got into the truck and started the motor. It strained and coughed. Connie felt Dooley shake a little. She held her breath.

Slowly, slowly, Dad moved the truck forward, pulling Dooley out of the crevasse. Finally, the mammoth set one front foot and then the other onto solid ice. When he pulled himself out he did a little shake to throw all the little ice splinters out of his hairs.

"So long," Dad called, unlocking the chain from around Dooley, rolling it up, and tossing it into the back of the pickup. He got in, waved through the window, and drove off.

"Unreal," said Connie.

"I don't know whether it's real or not," Dooley said, "but you're really lucky. You have so many people to help you."

"I guess I do, but what about you? Don't you have friends?"

"Sure. There's a whole herd of woolly mammoths over the next snow bank, and one of them is pretty too. But I've never talked to her."

"Why ever not?"

"I don't look good enough. I have so much matted hair."

"My mom could make you look terrific."

What did you have in mind?"

Deanna, Connie's mom, was standing next to Dooley, clutching the collar of her old blue winter coat around her neck, and holding her pink case with all the combs and brushes.

"Mom! Connie shouted. "What are you doing here? Never mind. I know. You're here because I said I needed you."

"You got it," Mom said. "Now, what seems to be wrong?"

"Dooley doesn't like his hair."

"No problem." Mom took out a comb as big as a rake. She walked all around Dooley, raking the comb through the long matted hairs.

When she was done, his hair was so smooth, the ends curled. Then Connie's mom squirted some sweet smelling stuff on each of Dooley's four knees. "I can't reach behind your ears," she said.

"But, Mom," Connie tried to whisper from way up on

Dooley's back, "he's a guy.

"Don't worry. It's your father's after shave," she called up brightly.

Dooley was so happy he wanted to lift Connie's mom up onto his back too, but when he curled his trunk around her, poof! She disappeared.

"Doesn't your family ever stick around?" he asked.

"Sure," she replied, laughing.

"Now, hang on tight," Dooley shouted, "We're off to meet Julie."

"Her name is Julie?"

"Sure. If I married her, we could be Dooley and Julie Woolly."

Connie clapped her hands and laughed out loud. When Dooley started to run, she didn't have time to grab onto his hair.

"Stop shaking!" Connie called. But it was too late. The running and shaking went on, and Connie slipped off Dooley's back.

In the distance she saw him bounding ahead happily, not realizing that Connie wasn't on his back anymore.

She opened her eyes. Mom and Dad were there, shaking the bed.

"Gee, thanks," she said. "Both of you really came through for me."

Mom and Dad just looked at each other. Then Dad said, "Time to get up, Connie. You're going to help me clean out the storage room today, remember?"

Connie smiled the widest smile she'd had in weeks. "And I thought nothing would ever be real around here again," she said.

The Magic Pie

by Marcia Levine Mazur

"Happy New Year to me, Happy New Year to me." Art whistled this to the tune of "Happy Birthday" as he opened the door and let his dog, Shereena, out into the yard.

Then he opened the refrigerator and poked his head inside. He was thinking of the story his teacher had told them about a genie who lived in a refrigerator.

The story had been exciting, but life seemed pretty dull right now. There wasn't even anything special in the fridge. Just some fruit, carrots scraped and ready to eat, stalks of celery, and a head of lettuce. He even found fresh fish wrapped in shiny white paper. Ugh.

Then he saw the pumpkin pie. It was the one Mom had made for Aunt Sarah's open house. Aunt Sarah always had an open house on New Year's Day, and Mom always made a pie for it. Art used to eat gobs of the pie until they found out he had diabetes. Now he just ate one piece.

But this morning he wanted more, lots more. It was New Year's Day, after all. Why couldn't he have all the foods he used to gobble down before he got diabetes?

Still thinking about the story, he put his right index fin-

180

ger on top of the pie and said out loud, "I wish I ate only sweets and stuff. And I wish they didn't make my blood sugar go up a single number."

The refrigerator light blinked three times! A wind whistled between the shelves! Art shivered and slammed the door.

Then he inched it open and peeked inside. Everything looked normal. Slowly, he took a carrot and bit off a chunk. It didn't crunch. Maybe it's spoiled, he thought.

He pulled it out of his mouth. It wasn't spoiled. The part he'd bitten off had turned to chocolate, but the part in his hand was still carrot! Art was so startled he swallowed the whole piece of chocolate. Delicious.

He took another bite. It happened again. The piece in his mouth turned to chocolate; the rest was still carrot.

Neat, he thought.

Next he chose a big red apple and bit into that. It tasted like a jelly doughnut. Jerking it out of his mouth, he stared at it. Yup. Still an apple. But the part he had chomped off had turned into a doughnut.

Art began to see what was happening. When food touched his lips it turned into something he liked. Terrific!

As he bit into a cracker, he thought, I wonder what will happen to this? Suddenly he was chewing a cherry jelly bean. He took another cracker, and then another. Each cracker became a different flavor jelly bean.

What a feast!

Art's mouth felt sticky after so many sweets, so he hurried to the bathroom, grabbed his blue toothbrush, and spread a glob of paste on it. But when he began to brush, the bristles turned to ice cream. Quickly, he washed them down the drain.

This wasn't fun any more. In fact, it was getting scary. He didn't want ice cream toothbrushes and chocolate carrots and doughnut apples and jelly bean crackers. He wanted real food and a real toothbrush.

Art began to feel sick. The sweets in his stomach seemed to be fighting each other, and he headed for his bedroom, shut the door, and fell onto his bed. Good thing Mom and Dad aren't up yet, he thought. He didn't want them to know about the silly wish and everything that was happening because of it.

Or was it happening? Maybe he was imagining it.

Let's see about my blood glucose. That was part of the wish, too, he thought. He tested his glucose. He was surprised that it was fine.

So the wish had come true. And now he had to find a way to stop it.

I know. I'll make another wish, he decided. Art stood and raised his right hand. He spoke out loud, "I wish the wish would be over and that everything would be the same again."

Nothing happened. No lights blinked. No wind blew.

Test it, he thought.

He fumbled for a stick of sugarless gum in his school bag, stuck the whole piece into his mouth, and chomped down on it. The gum crunched! It had turned into a potato chip. The new wish hadn't worked.

He lay back down again feeling miserable and listening to Shereena barking outside. She probably wanted to play. But what if she licked him on the mouth? Her tongue might turn into a slab of taffy.

A glass of cold water would sure taste good now, he thought. But what if the water turned to cherry soda when he drank it? He moaned.

Then he heard someone knocking on his door. "May I come in?" Oh no, it was Mom.

"I guess so."

She opened his door, walked to the bed, and lowered herself gently onto the side. "Don't you feel well?"

"I just want to rest."

"Have you checked your glucose?"

"It's fine."

"Could we take another look?"

"Sure." She watched as he checked it again. Still fine.

Then she did the one thing Art had been afraid of. She held her cheek out for him to kiss. "No!" He rolled over quickly. "I can't."

"So you think you're too old to kiss your mother?" He could see how hurt she was, but he couldn't tell her that if he kissed her cheek it might turn into candy or ice cream or something.

She hurried out and closed the door behind her. Art felt awful.

He sat up again. It was time to do some real thinking. Why had the wish worked this morning?

Well, first, he'd been alone. Second, he'd opened the refrigerator. Third, he'd touched the pumpkin pie. Fourth, he'd made the wish out loud.

He thought again about the story of the genie in the refrigerator. He didn't believe it, of course, but still. . . .

He knew what he had to do. Get into the kitchen alone, open the fridge, touch that pie, and take back the wish. And hurry. They'd all be leaving for the open house soon.

For a split second he pictured himself in Aunt Sarah's living room. There was a plate of food on his lap. And every bite he took turned into chocolate or ice cream or jelly beans. And everyone, especially Mom and Dad, was pointing and staring at him.

"Get moving," he ordered himself. Except that Mom was in the kitchen now. What should he do?

Shereena's barking gave him a plan. He would let her in the front door. She would run into the living room. Mom would rush out of the kitchen to get the dog out of the living room. That would give Art a minute alone in the kitchen, long enough to touch the pie.

"Here, Shereena," he called from the front door. "Here, girl." She bounded inside and, just as he planned, ran yelping all over the living room. Sure enough, Mom came running to get her out.

Art hopped into the kitchen and jerked the refrigerator door open. But before he could touch the pie, Mom and Shereena were there too.

"Back to square one," he thought.

Now he had another idea. Mom was still in her housecoat. He would wait right here until she left the kitchen to get dressed.

But it seemed she'd never leave. She put a roll of towels in the holder, stacked dishes, wiped the table, even opened a new bottle of soap. He drummed his hands on the sink.

Finally, she walked out.

Art rushed to the refrigerator, yanked the door open, and touched the pie.

"Hi, son. Ready to go?" Dad strolled in buttoning his shirt. Art felt like a balloon with the air let out.

"Sure," he said.

"Want a bite?" Dad opened the fridge and took out an

apple.

"No!" Art blocked his face with his arms as if he were fighting a vampire. Dad gave him a funny look.

Then Mom was back, taking the pie out of the refrigerator, wrapping it in foil with Art watching in horror as if his life were being wrapped up too.

"I'll carry it," he said quickly. She handed him the pie and he followed them out the door.

Mom and Dad got into the front seat of the car. Art slipped into the back, the pie on his lap.

But when Dad started the motor, Art started to panic. They would go to the party. Everyone would eat the pie. It would be gone, and he would never ever get to take his wish back! Nothing in his life would ever be the same again.

"Wait," he called. "I forgot something important."

"What?"

He couldn't think of a single thing he might have forgotten. There wouldn't be anyone at Aunt Sarah's to show his baseball cards or mitt to. He didn't even have a new jacket or boots to show off.

Then his stomach gave a twinge from the chocolate carrot, the doughnut apple, the jelly bean crackers, and the ice cream toothbrush.

"Shereena!" he shouted. "I forgot to let Shereena out." He opened the door and jumped out of the car.

"Art, you're still holding the pie!" Mom shouted. "Leave the pie!"

But Art was already unlocking the door, the pie cradled in his arm.

Finally alone in the kitchen, Art yanked the fridge open, set the pie on a shelf, snatched the foil off, stuck his finger on top, and shouted, "I wish my wish never happened. I wish everything would be the way it was."

The lights blinked. The breeze blew. Art shivered. Whew! I did it, he thought to himself.

Just to make sure, he bit into a carrot. It crunched loudly. He bit again. It crunched again. "Whoopeee!" he shouted.

Art was so relieved he ran back to the car still holding the carrot, but forgetting the pie and Shereena.

Mom and Dad were staring at him. "For Heaven's sake, where's the pie?" Mom asked. "And what in the world are you doing with a carrot?"

Art took another big crunchy bite and chewed and chewed it with his eyes closed. "Don't you think a crunchy carrot is the sweetest sound in the world?" he asked.

Mom and Dad looked at each other and just shook their heads.